T0181992

IFIP Advances in Information and Communication Technology **616**

Editor-in-Chief

Kai Rannenberg, Goethe University Frankfurt, Germany

IFIP – The International Federation for Information Processing

IFIP was founded in 1960 under the auspices of UNESCO, following the first World Computer Congress held in Paris the previous year. A federation for societies working in information processing, IFIP's aim is two-fold: to support information processing in the countries of its members and to encourage technology transfer to developing nations. As its mission statement clearly states:

IFIP is the global non-profit federation of societies of ICT professionals that aims at achieving a worldwide professional and socially responsible development and application of information and communication technologies.

IFIP is a non-profit-making organization, run almost solely by 2500 volunteers. It operates through a number of technical committees and working groups, which organize events and publications. IFIP's events range from large international open conferences to working conferences and local seminars.

The flagship event is the IFIP World Computer Congress, at which both invited and contributed papers are presented. Contributed papers are rigorously refereed and the rejection rate is high.

As with the Congress, participation in the open conferences is open to all and papers may be invited or submitted. Again, submitted papers are stringently refereed.

The working conferences are structured differently. They are usually run by a working group and attendance is generally smaller and occasionally by invitation only. Their purpose is to create an atmosphere conducive to innovation and development. Refereeing is also rigorous and papers are subjected to extensive group discussion.

Publications arising from IFIP events vary. The papers presented at the IFIP World Computer Congress and at open conferences are published as conference proceedings, while the results of the working conferences are often published as collections of selected and edited papers.

IFIP distinguishes three types of institutional membership: Country Representative Members, Members at Large, and Associate Members. The type of organization that can apply for membership is a wide variety and includes national or international societies of individual computer scientists/ICT professionals, associations or federations of such societies, government institutions/government related organizations, national or international research institutes or consortia, universities, academies of sciences, companies, national or international associations or federations of companies.

More information about this series at http://www.springer.com/series/6102

Aleksander Byrski · Tadeusz Czachórski ·
Erol Gelenbe · Krzysztof Grochla ·
Yuko Murayama (Eds.)

Computer Science Protecting Human Society Against Epidemics

First IFIP TC 5 International Conference, ANTICOVID 2021
Virtual Event, June 28–29, 2021
Revised Selected Papers

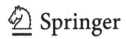 Springer

Editors
Aleksander Byrski (iD)
AGH University of Science and Technology
Kraków, Poland

Erol Gelenbe (iD)
Institute of Theoretical and Applied
Informatics, Polish Academy of Sciences
Gliwice, Poland

Yuko Murayama (iD)
Tsuda University
Tokyo, Japan

Tadeusz Czachórski (iD)
Institute of Theoretical and Applied
Informatics, Polish Academy of Sciences
Gliwice, Poland

Krzysztof Grochla (iD)
Institute of Theoretical and Applied
Informatics, Polish Academy of Sciences
Gliwice, Poland

ISSN 1868-4238   ISSN 1868-422X (electronic)
IFIP Advances in Information and Communication Technology
ISBN 978-3-030-86584-9   ISBN 978-3-030-86582-5 (eBook)
https://doi.org/10.1007/978-3-030-86582-5

This Springer imprint is published by the registered company Springer Nature Switzerland AG
The registered company address is: Gewerbestrasse 11, 6330 Cham, Switzerland

Preface

The COVID-19 pandemic concerns everyone. Therefore, in this volume we present the proceedings of the working conference on "Computer Science Protecting Human Society Against Epidemics" that was held online during June 28–29, 2021. The proposal for the event emanated from the Committee on Informatics of the Polish Academy of Sciences (which is an IFIP member) and was sustained by Technical Committee 5 of IFIP on Information Technology Applications, and especially by its Working Group WG 5.15 Information Technology in Disaster Risk Reduction.

The main topics of the conference were announced as comprising the following:

- IT support for modeling and understanding the COVID-19 pandemic and its effects,
- IT aspects of social life during a pandemic, and
- Security and privacy during pandemics.

This volume contains the best 11 submissions (10 full articles and a work in progress) from authors in various countries in three continents, namely Bangladesh, Bulgaria, France, Kazakhstan, Latvia, Poland, Russia, Slovenia, UK, Ukraine, and the USA. Many of these papers are the outcome of international collaborations.

Even if the number of contributions in these proceedings is small, they concern a very large spectrum of problems, ranging from linguistics for automatic translation of medical terms to a proposition for a worldwide system of fast reaction to emerging pandemics. Some of the papers relate to mathematics and modeling, such as statistical problems related to death-rate computations and the use of information entropy in the analysis of pandemic waves viewed as stochastic time series. Some papers deal with numerical problems in epidemiological models, deep learning, and neural networks to forecast the spread of pandemics. Other papers discuss high-performance computing systems for fighting pandemics, monitoring virus spread, and bioinformatics for virus analysis. We also have an empirical study of the impact of pandemics on student life, and a study of journal attitudes towards pandemics.

We are very grateful to the authors of all submitted or accepted papers for their contributions. We also thank the keynote speaker who kindly accepted our invitation. Finally, we wish to thank the Program Committee members and the referees for their important contributions to these proceedings.

July 2021

Aleksander Byrski
Tadeusz Czachórski
Erol Gelenbe
Krzysztof Grochla
Yuko Murayama

Organization

General Chair

Yuko Murayama   Tsuda University, Japan

Program Committee Chairs

Aleksander Byrski   AGH University of Science and Technology, Poland
Tadeusz Czachórski   IITiS PAN, Poland
Erol Gelenbe   IITiS PAN, Poland
Krzysztof Grochla   IITiS PAN, Poland

Program Committee

Luis Soares Barbosa   UNU-EGOV and University of Minho, Portugal
Andrzej Bartoszewicz   Technical University of Lodz, Poland
Tadeusz Burczyński   Institute of Fundamental Technological Research PAS,
                                 Poland
Juan Burguillo-Rial   Universida de Vigo, Spain
Maria Carla Calzarossa   Universita di Pavia, Italy
Denis Cavalucci   INSA Strasbourg, France
Witold Charatonik   Wroclaw University, Poland
Carlos Cotta   Universidad de Málaga, Spain
Philippe Dallemagne   Centre Suisse d'Electronique et de Microtechnique,
                                 Switzerland
Ivanna Dronyuk   Lviv Polytechnic National University, Ukraine
Włodzislaw Duch   Nicolaus Copernicus University, Poland
Eduard Dundler   International Federation for Information Processing,
                                 Austria
Anna Fabijańska   Technical University of Lodz, Poland
Yuliya Gaidamaka   Peoples' Friendship University of Russia, Russia
Krzysztof Grochla   IITiT PAN, Poland
Aleksandra Gruca   Silesian University of Technology, Poland
Andres Iglesias   University of Cantabria, Spain
Szymon Jaroszewicz   Institute of Computer Science, Polish Academy
                                 of Sciences, Poland
Piotr Jędrzejowicz   Gdynia Maritime University, Poland
Miłosz Kadziński   Poznan University of Technology, Poland
Marek Kisiel-Dorohinicki   AGH University of Science and Technology, Poland
Józef Korbicz   University of Zielona Gora, Poland
Stanisław Kozielski   Silesian University of Technology, Poland
Krzysztof Kozłowski   Poznan University of Technology, Poland

Miroslaw Kutyłowski	Wroclaw University of Science and Technology, Poland
Tom Lenaerts	Université Libre de Bruxelles, Belgium
Daoliang Li	China Agricultural University, China
Jacek Mańdziuk	Warsaw University of Technology, Poland
Eunika Merciel-Laurent	Universite de Reims Champagne-Ardenne, France
Evsey Morozov	Institute of Applied Mathematical Research of the Karelian Research Centre, Russian Academy of Sciences, Russia
Zbigniew Nahorski	Systems Research Institute, Polish Academy of Sciences, Poland
Jerzy Nawrocki	Poznan University of Technology, Poland
Erich J. Neuhold	Universität Wien, Austria
Ngoc Thanh Nguyen	Wroclaw University of Science and Technology, Poland
Maciej Ogorzałek	AGH University of Science and Technology, Poland
Michele Pagano	University of Pisa, Italy
Philippe Palanque	Université Paul Sabatier, France
Wojciech Penczek	Institute of Computer Sciences, Polish Academy of Sciences, Poland
Joanna Polańska	Silesian University of Technology, Poland
Henryk Rybiński	Warsaw University of Technology, Poland
Manoj Sharma	Rustamji Institute of Technology, India
Miroslaw Skibniewski	University of Maryland, College Park, USA
Andrzej Skowron	Warsaw University, Poland
Dominik Slęzak	Warsaw University, Poland
Roman Slowiński	Poznan University of Technology, Poland
Tomasz Szmuc	AGH University of Science and Technology, Poland
Dimiter Velev	University of National and World Economy, Bulgaria
Józef Woźniak	Politechnika Gdańska, Poland
Michał Woźniak	Wroclaw University of Technology, Poland
Robert Wrembel	Poznan University of Technology, Poland
Roman Wyrzykowski	Czestochowa University of Technology, Poland
Juan Burguillo Rial	University of Vigo, Spain
Sławomir Zadrożny	Systems Research Institute, Polish Academy of Sciences, Poland
Plamena Zlateva	Institute of Robotics, Bulgarian Academy of Sciences, Bulgaria

Contents

Bioinformatic and MD Analysis of N501Y SARS-CoV-2 (UK) Variant

Marko Jukić[1,2](✉) iD, Sebastjan Kralj[1], Natalia Nikitina[3] iD,
and Urban Bren[1,2](✉)

[1] Faculty of Chemistry and Chemical Engineering, Laboratory of Physical Chemistry
and Chemical Thermodynamics, University of Maribor,
Smetanova ulica 17, 2000 Maribor, Slovenia
{marko.jukic,urban.bren}@um.si
[2] Faculty of Mathematics, Natural Sciences and Information Technologies,
University of Primorska, Glagoljaška 8, 6000 Koper, Slovenia
[3] Research Center of the Russian Academy of Sciences, Institute of Applied
Mathematical Research, Karelian, Pushkinskaya 11, 185910 Petrozavodsk, Russia

Abstract. COVID-19 is a disease caused by severe acute respiratory
syndrome coronavirus 2 or SARS-CoV-2 pathogen. Although a number
of new vaccines are available to combat this threat, a high prevalence
of novel mutant viral variants is observed in all world regions affected
by this infection. Among viral proteomes, the highly glycosylated spike
protein (Sprot) of SARS-CoV-2 has received the most attention due to
its interaction with the host receptor ACE2. To understand the mechanisms of viral variant infectivity and the interaction of the RBD of Sprot
with the host ACE2, we performed a large-scale mutagenesis study of
the RBD-ACE2 interface by performing 1780 point mutations *in silico* and identifying the ambiguous stabilisation of the interface by the
most common point mutations described in the literature. Furthermore,
we pinpointed the N501Y mutation at the RBD of Sprot as profoundly
affecting complex formation and confirmed greater stability of the N501Y
mutant compared to wild-type (WT) viral S protein by molecular dynamics experiments. These findings could be important for the study and
design of upcoming vaccines, PPI inhibitor molecules, and therapeutic
antibodies or antibody mimics.

Keywords: COVID-19 · SARS-CoV-2 · Point mutation ·
SARS-CoV-2 variants · Protein-protein interactions · Drug design

Abbreviations

ACE2 Angiotensin-converting enzyme 2

Supported by the Slovenian Ministry of Science and Education infrastructure project
grant HPC-RIVR, by the Slovenian Research Agency (ARRS) programme and project
grants P2-0046 and J1-2471, and by Slovenian Ministry of Education, Science and
Sports programme grant OP20.04342.

© IFIP International Federation for Information Processing 2021
Published by Springer Nature Switzerland AG 2021
A. Byrski et al. (Eds.): ANTICOVID 2021, IFIP AICT 616, pp. 1–13, 2021.
https://doi.org/10.1007/978-3-030-86582-5_1

MD Molecular Dynamics
PDB Protein Data Bank
PPI Protein-Protein Interactions
RBD Receptor Binding Domain
WHO World Health Organisation

1 Introduction

In 1962, scientists isolated a new group of viruses that cause cold (enveloped positive-sense single-stranded (+ssRNA) RNA virus). They named this new group of viruses, *coronaviruses* after their characteristic morphological appearance, namely they are named after crown spikes located on their surface [9].

The viruses from the *Coronaviridae* family have rarely attracted attention over the last half-century. The first example was in 2003, when the coronavirus caused an outbreak of SARS (Severe Acute Respiratory Syndrome; pathogen virus named SARS-CoV) in mainland China and Hong Kong. Another example was in 2012 when the Middle East coronavirus of the respiratory syndrome (MERS-CoV) led to an outbreak of the Middle East respiratory syndrome (MERS) in Saudi Arabia mainland China and the United Arab Emirates and the Republic of Korea [12, 16, 26].

In late 2019, SARS-CoV-2, a member of the *Coronaviridae* family, appeared in Wuhan, China, and a creeping spread among the human population has begun [39]. The WHO declared a pandemic on 11 March 2020 [14, 25]. At the time of writing this article, the COVID-19 disease (caused by SARS-CoV-2) has spread rapidly worldwide, claiming more than **3** million lives (https://www.worldo\discretionary-me\discretionary-ters.info/coronavirus/coronavirus-death-toll/). As the SARS-CoV-2 virus has become a critical health problem, scientists immediately began research to clarify the virus' mode of action [36]. COVID-19 disease is of grave global concern because, while the majority of cases displays mild symptoms, a variable percentage (0.2 to >5%!) of patients progresses to pneumonia and multi-organ failure leading to potential death, especially without medical assistance [13, 27, 31].

As of now, we have registered vaccines against SARS-CoV-2 [1, 7], but still no antivirals and only a few of therapeutic options for COVID-19 treatment [23, 28]. As vaccines represent the flagship in the fight against COVID-19 pandemic, high viral mutation rate can translate to changes in the structures of key viral proteins rendering available vaccines ineffective [30].

In late 2020, new SARS-CoV-2 variants was reported; mainly B.1.1.7 variant (UK variant, named alpha by WHO as of 7th June, 2021; https://www.who.int/) and B.1.351 variant (beta) or South African variant [33, 35]. Both variants carry N501Y mutation in the RBD (receptor binding domain) of the Sprot (spike protein) that is associated with increased viral transmission [11]. The South African variant carries K417N and E484K mutations in the Sprot that are potentially responsible for the diminished binding of viral Sprot to host antibodies [38]. In Brazil, P.1 (gamma) variant with known N501Y, E484K and novel K417T mutation was reported [10].

In early 2021, a novel SARS-CoV-2 variant B.1.617 (delta) nicknamed "the double mutant" or Indian variant was reported causing infections in India and slowly spreading all over the world via global travel practices [6,8,29,40]. Acquired key mutations in S protein, especially at the receptor binding domain (RBD) are under investigation (delta plus) due to potential of greater infectivity, transmissibility, or even the potential to escape host immune responses [34]. Summary of main SARS-CoV-2 variants is provided in Table 1. To this end, we sought to investigate a staple **N501Y** mutation on RBD binding domain present in B.1.1.7, B.1.351 and P.1 variants via FoldX mutational scan, molecular dynamic (MD) analysis and compare it to wild type.

Table 1. Summary of SARS-CoV-2 variants

Variant[a]	Alternative name	Sprot/all mutations	Key mutations	Comment
B.1.1.7	UK Variant-alpha	8/23	E69/70 del 144Y del **N501Y** (RBD) A570D P681H	Higher transmissibility
B.1.351	South African Variant-beta	9/21	K417N (RBD) E484K (RBD) **N501Y** (RBD) orf1b del	Escape host immune response
P.1	Brasil Variant-gamma	10/17	K417N/T (RBD) E484K (RBD) **N501Y** (RBD) orf1b del	Under research
B.1.617	Indian Variant-delta	7/23	G142D delta156-157/R158G. A222V **L452R** (RBD) **T478K** (RBD) D614G P681R D950N	Under research

[a] Other known variants are COH.20G, S Q677H (Midwest variant) and L452R, B1429; reference https://www.uniprot.org/uniprot/P0DTC.

2   Methods and Results

2.1   FoldX Calculations – Mutagenesis Study

FoldX relative free energies ($\Delta\Delta G$) for Spro RBD mutants were calculated using FoldX, version 5 [5]. To analyse the influence of the FoldX point mutations along with FoldX optimisation, 3D structures of wild type along with FoldX mutants were iteratively used for $\Delta\Delta G$ prediction. Point mutations were performed using the `--command=BuildModel` switch and supplied individual_list.txt file with `--mutant-file` switch. Number of runs was set at default value of 5. All other options were set to default, including temperature (298 K), ionic strength (0.05 M), and pH (7), VdWDesign 2 strong, clashCapDesign 5, backBoneAtoms false, dipoles true and complexClashes parameter set to 1. *Inhouse* script was prepared to calculate all possible mutations of RBD binding domain of SARS-CoV-2 S protein (PDB ID: 6M0J) with sequence from K417 towards Y505 (length of 89) for a total of 1780 point mutations (Table 2).

Table 2. Sequences used for mutagenesis study

Spike protein length	229

>6M0J_2—Chain E—Spike protein S1—Severe acute respiratory syndrome coronavirus 2 (2697049)
RVQPTESIVRFPNITNLCPFGEVFNATRFASVYAWNRKRISNCVADYSVLYN SASFSTFKCYGVSPTKLNDLCFTNVYADSFVIRGDEVRQIAPGQTG**KIADY NYKLPDDFTGCVIAWNSNNLDSKVGGNYNYLYRLFRKSNLKPFE RDISTEIYQAGSTPCNGVEGFNCYFPLQSYGFQPTNGVGY**QPYRV VVLSFELLHAPATVCGPKKSTNLVKNKCVNFHHHHHH

Mutagenesis study sequence (RBD) length89
KIADYNYKLPDDFTGCVIAWNSNNLDSKVGGNYNYLYRLFRKSNLKPFERD ISTEIYQAGSTPCNGVEGFNCYFPLQSYGFQPTNGVGY

In the mutagenesis study, individual point mutation calculations were repeated once and mutations with no structural change left for validation purposes where all no-change mutation produced $\Delta\Delta G$ energies below 0.1 kcal/mol.

2.2 Model Preparation

The 2.45 Å crystal structure (PDB ID: 6M0J) of SARS-CoV-2 spike receptor-binding domain bound with ACE2 was obtained via RCSB PDB Database [21]. Chain E (Spike protein S1) was chosen for further work where analysis of protein-protein interaction (PPI) with chain A (Angiotensin-converting enzyme 2) was conducted. Complex was prepared Yasara STRUCTURE (19.6.6.L.64) software [20]. Missing hydrogens were added, missing bonds and bond orders set, overlapping atoms adjusted, rebuild side-chains with missing atoms, hydrogen bonds optimized, proteins capped (Ace, Nma) and residue ionisation assigned at $pH = 7.4$ [18,19].

The interface of Sprot RBD domain in up(open) conformation was referenced against SARS-CoV-2 S trimer, S-open complex (PDB ID: 7DK3) where superimposition of chain E from 6M0J and chain C from 7DK3 with an all atom RMSD of 1.429 Å produced a nearly similar conformation of S protein RBD. Carbohydrates were not considered in the vicinity of RBD interface (Fig. 1).

2.3 Molecular Dynamics

We performed MD simulations of the chimeric receptor-binding domain (RBD) of the SARS-CoV-2 spike protein bound to the human Angiotensin-converting enzyme 2 (ACE2) to study the effect of mutational changes to binding dynamics of the protein complex. The simulation inputs were prepared using the

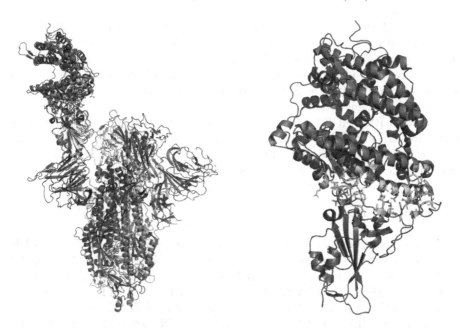

Fig. 1. Left: 7dk3 with S protein chains A B and C colored red, orange and yellow respectively and superimposed 6m0j colored magenta. Right: 6m0j complex where chain A (ACE2) is colored magenta, chain E (RBD) colored blue and PPI interface emphasized in green color. All models are depicted with ribbon presentation (Color figure online).

CHARMM-GUI web interface for the CHARMM biomolecular simulations program [4,15]. The input structure PDB ID: 6VW1 was chosen among the many RBD-ACE2 structures due to its superior resolution and high scoring percentile ranks provided by the web interface of PDB [32].

Using the CHARMM-GUI server, we generated an additional mutant N501 using the built-in functionality. The mutation was chosen due to the ever-increasing prevalence which may indicate that this mutation, occurring in the RBD binding site increases affinity for the host ACE2 [3]. Glycans present in the structure were removed beforehand since they were not present in the interaction site and would increase computing time. Both protein structures were solvated using TIP3P water and neutralized using Na^+ and Cl^- ions (0.1M) to approximate physiological conditions. To remove existing atomic clashes and optimization of the atomic geometry, 50 steps of the steepest descent and 500 steps of adopted basis Newton-Raphson energy minimization was performed. The final step of equilibration was a 1 ns NVT molecular dynamics simulation during which the protein was heated to 310.15 K using the hoover heat bath with the integration time-step set to 1 fs.

Final molecular dynamics production runs were carried out using NPT ensemble with periodic boundary conditions applied, the time-step set to 2 fs and the thermostat set to 310.15 K. Non-bonded interaction cutoff was achieved using a force-based switching function between 12 and 16Å. Bonds to hydrogens were constrained using the SHAKE algorithm. The CHARMM36m force field was used for all simulations.

For both RBD-ACE2 structures the production runs were generated using GPU acceleration with the final analysis performed on the last 180 ns of the production run, with the first 20 ns of the production runs ignored in order to minimize the error arising from different initial velocity seeds.

3   Discussion

Structural inspection and superimposition of complexes of Sprot-ACE2 (PDB ID: 6M0J) and Sprot open conformation (PDB ID: 7DK3) the Sprot RBD-ACE2 PPI interface was identified and key RBD residues in contact with ACE2 defined as following: 417 LYS, 445 VAL, 446 GLY, 449 TYR, 453 TYR, 455 LEU, 456 PHE, 473 TYR, 475 ALA, 476 GLY, 484 GLU, 486 PHE, 487 ASN, 489 TYR, 493 GLN, 496 GLY, 498 GLN, 500 THR, 501 ASN, 502 GLY, 503 VAL, 505 TYR. Literature reported key mutations on this interface such as E484K - S African variant that could escape immune responses, Q493N or Q493Y with reduced host ACE2-binding affinity in vitro, N501Y UK and S African variant that influences virulence or N501T with reduced host ACE2-binding affinity in vitro all according to P0DTC2 Uniprot reference.

Lately, two key mutations L452R and E484Q from Indian variant are under investigation [8]. We conducted a full RBD 417-505 mutagenesis study using FoldX in order to asses these key mutations and their effect on the stability of the system, in total 1780 point mutations (Fig. 2) [42].

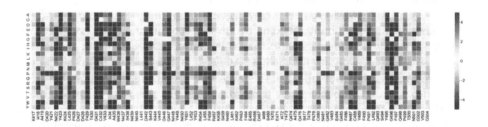

Fig. 2. Complete RBD-ACE2 interface mutagenesis heatmap where deep green color indicates positive FoldX force field Δ energies (destabilising) and deep purple contrasting positive FoldX force field Δ energies (stabilising).

We observed FoldX total energies of 0.374201, 0.622215 and −0.950612 kcal/mol upon point mutations E484K, Q493N and Q493Y respectively. All mutations are postulated as non-significantly influencing the stability of RBD-ACE2 complex. Literature reports on reduced binding affinity towards ACE2 but our preliminary results indicate the complex formation is more complex than initially postulated [17]. Indeed, the literature corroborates our observations [37].

Furthermore, L452R and E484Q point mutations from Indian viral variant display insignificant FoldX force field Δ energies of 0.0424621, 0.0912967 kcal/mol, respectively [2,24,41]. On the contrary, FoldX force field Δ energies of 6.18517 and −0.449581 kcal/mol were observed for UK variant point mutations N501Y and N501T, respectively, indicating a predictable effect of N501Y point mutation of RBD-ACE2 binding, an observation confirmed by experimental evaluation [22].

In order to further assess the influence of N501Y point mutation, we conducted a molecular dynamics (MD) experiment on WT RBD-ACE2 and N501Y mutated protein (Figs. 3, 4, 5 and 6).

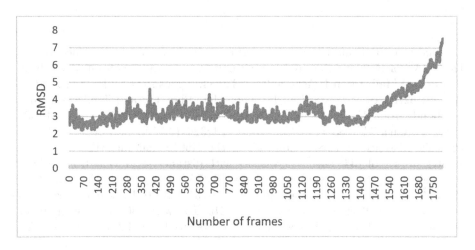

Fig. 3. Root mean square deviation of wild type RBD-ACE2 complex through simulation time

From the 180 ns production runs, it can be observed the point mutated N501Y RBD-ACE2 complex displays comparable conformational stability all along the production run with backbone RMSD of 3.37 ± 0.85Å and radius of gyration $31, 69 \pm 0.48$Å versus $2.87 \pm 0, 26$Å and radius of gyration of 31.30 ± 0.22Å for WT, respectively. Nevertheless, after the inflection point at 140 ns, the WT experiences a conformational change leading to a linear increase of both measured parameters. The amino acid contact profiles are also distinct as can be observed in Table 3 and 4 where residues with longest contact times at the interface are tabulated.

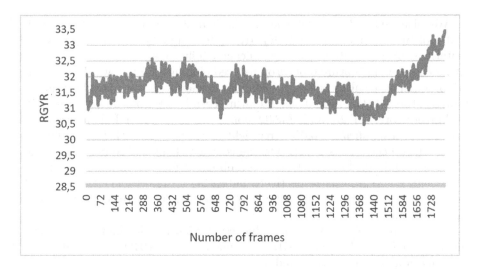

Fig. 4. Radius of Gyration of the wild type RBD-ACE2 complex through simulation time

Wild type RBD after the MD experiment displays a contact surface area of 1126.88Å^2 for RBD interface residues with distance $< 5\text{Å}$ away from ACE2, from that 64.37Å^2 falls towards Asp and Glu, $329{,}84\text{Å}^2$ goes to Ser, Thr, Asn and Gln and $597{,}62\text{Å}^2$ towards Ala, Val, Ile, Leu, Met, Phe, Tyr and Trp. Key hydrogen bonds from RBD towards ACE2 are Tyr449-Glu37 (1.88Å), Glu484-Lys31 (1.88Å), Asn487-Tyr83 (2.04Å), Thr500-Gly326 (2.15Å) and Asn501-Gly354 with the distance of 1.98Å. Contrasting the N501Y mutant RBD displays a greater surface of 1348.94Å^2 for residues with distance $< 5\text{Å}$ away from ACE2.

Analogously to WT surface analyses 73.35Å^2 falls towards Asp and Glu, 292.17Å^2 goes to Ser, Thr, Asn and Gln and 731.91Å^2 to hydrophobic residues with additional effective contacts via Arg, His, Lys with 130.04Å^2. In the point mutant following key hydrogen bonds are observed: Arg439-Gln325 (1.88Å),

Table 3. Amino-acid residues with the longest time in contact during simulations for N501Y RBD.

RBD residue ID	ACE2 residue ID	Total time in contact (ps)
Tyr501	Lys353	5876
Tyr473	Glu23	455
Ala475	Ser19	272
Ala475	Gln24	361
Asn487	Tyr83	1306
Tyr489	Tyr83	541
Thr500	Asp355	412

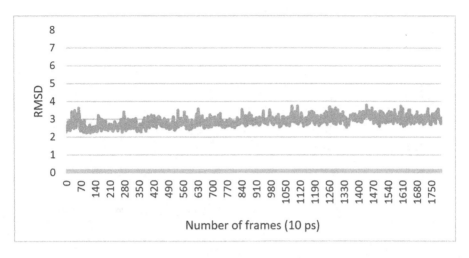

Fig. 5. Root mean square deviation of N501Y mutated RBD-ACE2 complex through simulation time

Table 4. Amino-acid residues with the longest time in contact during simulations for wild type RBD.

RBD residue ID	ACE2 residue ID	Total time in contact (ps)
Thr446	Lys353	550
Tyr449	Asp38	826
Asn487	Tyr83	2285
Tyr489	Tyr83	1100
Ser494	Hsd34	400
Gln498	Tyr41	450
Val503	Gln325	300

Asn487-Tyr83 (1.78Å), Thr500-Asp355 (1.87Å) and Gly502-Lys353 with distance of 1.82Å. It is evident the bulky tyrosine at position 501 effectively increases the contact area and optimises the interface interaction profile towards more hydrophobic contacts and conservation of hydrogen bond propensity (Fig. 7).

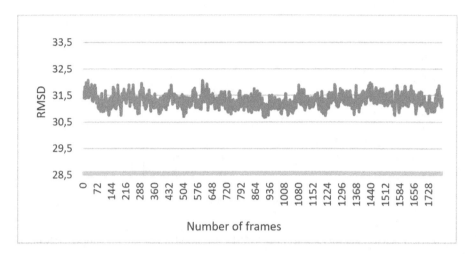

Fig. 6. Radius of gyration of the N501Y mutant RBD-ACE2 complex through simulation time

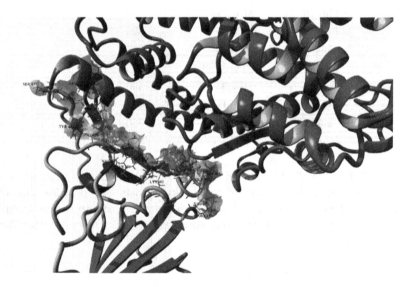

Fig. 7. Sprot RBD-host ACE2 interface for N501Y point mutant. Proteins are depicted in cartoon model representation ACE2 colored blue and RBD in red, green, blue, cyan color with interacting residues in line model, labelled with mutated residue N501Y emphasized as ball and stick model colored green. Surface area of interacting RBD is presented in gray color (Color figure online).

4   Conclusions

In 1962, scientists isolated a new group of viruses that cause colds - enveloped positive-sense single-stranded; +ssRNA; RNA viruses. They named this new group of viruses, coronaviruses after their characteristic spikes on their surface. In late 2019/early 2020, a global pandemic was declared by WHO and the new pathogen named SARS-CoV-2 from the *Coronaviridae* family was quickly and effectively sequenced and described. Following the introduction of vaccines against the new pathogen, a wide range of viral variants were thoroughly investigated, particularly with regard to vaccine efficacy. To analyze the key profile of the viral Sprot RBD - host ACE2 interaction, we first performed a large-scale mutagenesis study of the RBD-ACE2 interface using FoldX software, where we performed 1780 point mutations *in silico* and identified the ambiguous stabilization of the interface by the most frequent point mutations described in the literature. Indeed, this interface was difficult to quantify under the FoldX force field, but we still identified a profound impact on RBD-ACE2 by the point mutation N501Y. In MD analysis, we confirmed greater stability and enlarged contact area of the N501Y mutant compared to the wild-type (WT) viral S protein. These findings could be of great value for the study and design of upcoming vaccines, PPI inhibitor molecules and therapeutic antibodies or antibody mimics.

Acknowledgements. We thank Javier Delgado Blanco and Luis Serrano Pubul from FoldX for their support. Heartfelt thanks to Črtomir Podlipnik, a friend and a scientific colleague.

*Thank You, participants in the COVID.SI community (*www.co-vid.si *and* www.sidock.si*) for supporting our work. Thank You All!*

Conflicts of Interest. The authors declare no conflict of interest.

References

1. Amanat, F., Krammer, F.: SARS-CoV-2 vaccines: status report. Immunity **52**(4), 583–589 (2020)
2. Banu, S., et al.: A distinct phylogenetic cluster of Indian severe acute respiratory syndrome coronavirus 2 isolates. Open Forum Infect. Dis. **7**(11), ofaa434 (2020)
3. Bracken, C.J., et al.: Bi-paratopic and multivalent VH domains block ACE2 binding and neutralize SARS-CoV-2. Nat. Chem. Biol. **17**(1), 113–121 (2021)
4. Brooks, B.R., et al.: CHARMM: the biomolecular simulation program. J. Comput. Chem. **30**(10), 1545–1614 (2009)
5. Buß, O., Rudat, J., Ochsenreither, K.: FoldX as protein engineering tool: better than random based approaches? Comput. Struct. Biotechnol. J. **16**, 25–33 (2018)
6. Chatterjee, P.: Covid-19: India authorises Sputnik V vaccine as cases soar to more than 180 000 a day BMJ **373**, 978 (2021)
7. Chen, W.H., Strych, U., Hotez, P.J., Bottazzi, M.E.: The SARS-CoV-2 vaccine pipeline: an overview. Curr. Trop. Med. Rep. **7**(2), 61–64 (2020)
8. Cherian, S., et al.: Convergent evolution of SARS-CoV-2 spike mutations, L452R, E484Q and P681R, in the second wave of COVID-19 in Maharashtra, India. BioRxiv (2021)

9. De Wit, E., Van Doremalen, N., Falzarano, D., Munster, V.J.: SARS and MERS: recent insights into emerging coronaviruses. Nat. Rev. Microbiol. **14**(8), 523–534 (2016)

10. Faria, N.R., et al.: Genomic characterisation of an emergent SARS-CoV-2 lineage in Manaus: preliminary findings. Virological (2021)

11. Gu, H., et al.: Adaptation of SARS-CoV-2 in BALB/c mice for testing vaccine efficacy. Science **369**(6511), 1603–1607 (2020)

12. Hilgenfeld, R., Peiris, M.: From SARS to MERS: 10 years of research on highly pathogenic human coronaviruses. Antivir. Res. **100**(1), 286–295 (2013)

13. Hopkins, J.: Mortality analyses. https://coronavirus.jhu.edu/data/mortality

14. Hui, D.S., et al.: The continuing 2019-nCoV epidemic threat of novel coronaviruses to global health–The latest 2019 novel coronavirus outbreak in Wuhan, China. Int. J. Infect. Dis. **91**, 264–266 (2020)

15. Jo, S., Kim, T., Iyer, V.G., Im, W.: CHARMM-GUI: a web-based graphical user interface for CHARMM. J. Comput. Chem. **29**(11), 1859–1865 (2008)

16. Kahn, J.S., McIntosh, K.: History and recent advances in coronavirus discovery. Pediatr. Infect. Dis. J. **24**(11), S223–S227 (2005)

17. Khan, A., et al.: Higher infectivity of the SARS-CoV-2 new variants is associated with K417N/T, E484K, and N501Y mutants: an insight from structural data. J. Cell. Physiol. (2021)

18. Krieger, E., Dunbrack, R.L., Hooft, R.W., Krieger, B.: Assignment of protonation states in proteins and ligands: combining pK a prediction with hydrogen bonding network optimization. In: Baron, R. (eds.) Computational Drug Discovery and Design. Methods in Molecular Biology (Methods and Protocols), vol. 819, pp. 405–421. Springer, New York(2012). https://doi.org/10.1007/978-1-61779-465-0_25

19. Krieger, E., Nielsen, J.E., Spronk, C.A., Vriend, G.: Fast empirical pKa prediction by Ewald summation. J. Mol. Graph. Model. **25**(4), 481–486 (2006)

20. Krieger, E., Vriend, G.: New ways to boost molecular dynamics simulations. J. Comput. Chem. **36**(13), 996–1007 (2015)

21. Lan, J., et al.: Structure of the SARS-CoV-2 spike receptor-binding domain bound to the ACE2 receptor. Nature **581**(7807), 215–220 (2020)

22. Leung, K., Shum, M.H., Leung, G.M., Lam, T.T., Wu, J.T.: Early transmissibility assessment of the N501Y mutant strains of SARS-CoV-2 in the United Kingdom, October to November 2020. Eurosurveillance **26**(1), 2002106 (2021)

23. Li, H., Zhou, Y., Zhang, M., Wang, H., Zhao, Q., Liu, J.: Updated approaches against SARS-CoV-2. Antimicrob. Agent. Chemother. **64**(6), e00483 (2020)

24. Q, Li., et al.: The impact of mutations in SARS-CoV-2 spike on viral infectivity and antigenicity. Cell **182**(5), 1284–1294 (2020)

25. Li, Q., et al.: Early transmission dynamics in Wuhan, China, of novel coronavirus-infected pneumonia. New Engl. J. Med. **382**, 1199-1207 (2020)

26. Lu, G., Wang, Q., Gao, G.F.: Bat-to-human: spike features determining 'host jump'of coronaviruses SARS-CoV, MERS-CoV, and beyond. Trends Microbiol. **23**(8), 468–478 (2015)

27. Lu, R., et al.: Genomic characterisation and epidemiology of 2019 novel coronavirus: implications for virus origins and receptor binding. Lancet **395**(10224), 565–574 (2020)

28. McKee, D.L., Sternberg, A., Stange, U., Laufer, S., Naujokat, C.: Candidate drugs against SARS-CoV-2 and COVID-19. Pharmacol. Res. **157**, 104859 (2020)

29. Moelling, K.: Within-host and between-host evolution in SARS-CoV-2–new variant's source. Viruses **13**(5), 751 (2021)

30. Naqvi, A.A.T., et al.: Insights into SARS-CoV-2 genome, structure, evolution, pathogenesis and therapies: Structural genomics approach. Biochim. Biophys. Acta (BBA) Mol. Basis Dis. **1866**(10), 165878 (2020)
31. O'Driscoll, M., et al.: Age-specific mortality and immunity patterns of SARS-CoV-2. Nature **590**(7844), 140–145 (2021)
32. Shang, J., et al.: Structural basis of receptor recognition by SARS-CoV-2. Nature **581**(7807), 221–224 (2020)
33. Tegally, H., et al.: Emergence and rapid spread of a new severe acute respiratory syndrome-related coronavirus 2 (SARS-CoV-2) lineage with multiple spike mutations in South Africa. MedRxiv (2020)
34. Teng, S., Sobitan, A., Rhoades, R., Liu, D., Tang, Q.: Systemic effects of missense mutations on SARS-CoV-2 spike glycoprotein stability and receptor-binding affinity. Brief. Bioinform. **22**(2), 1239–1253 (2021)
35. Volz, E., et al.: Transmission of SARS-CoV-2 Lineage B. 1.1. 7 in England: Insights from linking epidemiological and genetic data. MedRxiv **2020**, 12 (2021)
36. Wang, C., Horby, P.W., Hayden, F.G., Gao, G.F.: A novel coronavirus outbreak of global health concern. Lancet **395**(10223), 470–473 (2020)
37. Wang, W.B., Liang, Y., Jin, Y.Q., Zhang, J., Su, J.G., Li, Q.M.: E484K mutation in SARS-CoV-2 RBD enhances binding affinity with hACE2 but reduces interactions with neutralizing antibodies and nanobodies: Binding free energy calculation studies. bioRxiv (2021)
38. Wibmer, C.K., et al.: SARS-CoV-2 501Y. V2 escapes neutralization by South African COVID-19 donor plasma. Nat. Med. **27**(4), 622–625 (2021)
39. Wu, F., et al.: A new coronavirus associated with human respiratory disease in china. Nature **579**(7798), 265–269 (2020)
40. Yadav, P., et al.: Neutralization of variant under investigation B. 1.617 with sera of BBV152 vaccinees. bioRxiv (2021)
41. Yadav, P.D., et al.: SARS CoV-2 variant B. 1.617. 1 is highly pathogenic in hamsters than B. 1 variant. bioRxiv (2021)
42. Zhang, Y., et al.: Mutagenesis study to disrupt electrostatic interactions on the twofold symmetry interface of Escherichia coli bacterioferritin. J. Biochem. **158**(6), 505–512 (2015)

Ensuring Interoperability of Laboratory Tests and Results: A Linguistic Approach for Mapping French Laboratory Terminologies with LOINC

Namrata Patel[1,2]([✉]) [ID], Yoann Abel[1], Fleur Brun[1], and Guilhem Mayoral[1]

[1] Onaos, Montpellier, France
{namrata.patel,yoann.abel,fleur.brun,guilhem.mayoral}@onaos.com
[2] Université Paul Valéry Montpellier 3, équipe AMIS, Montpellier, France
namrata.patel@univ-montp3.fr
http://www.onaos.com

Abstract. With the increasing use of electronic patient records, interoperability of patient-related data is of primary concern and international standards have been developed to assure compatibility between health data management systems. The present study is a first step in this direction for laboratory tests written in french, following the French government's impetus for providing national health records for patients. To address the linguistic complexities inherent to this task, we adopt a natural language processing (NLP) methodology . Our pilot case study shows that computational linguistic assistance in aligning terminologies makes it 3 times faster for domain experts. The significant difference in performance between the existing state of the art and our tool reflects the impact of addressing the linguistic challenges involved in the mapping process, especially in the multilingual context.

Keywords: LOINC · Terminology mapping · NLP

1 Background and Significance

Standardised terminologies are increasingly used for structuring computerised health data today [1,5,11], facilitating the semantic interoperability between IT systems that process Electronic Health Records (EHR) [16]. LOINC (Logical Observation Identifiers Names and Codes), along with SNOMED and RxNORM, is one of the three most widely used standardised terminologies [10]. This terminology ensures the unambiguous identification of laboratory exams as well as clinical and biometric observations such as those described in prescriptions for these exams. In France, the digital health agency has entrusted the maintenance of this terminology to a consortium comprising the Assistance Publique

© IFIP International Federation for Information Processing 2021
Published by Springer Nature Switzerland AG 2021
A. Byrski et al. (Eds.): ANTICOVID 2021, IFIP AICT 616, pp. 14–22, 2021.
https://doi.org/10.1007/978-3-030-86582-5_2

Hôpitaux de Paris (AP-HP), the companies Vidal and Mondeca, and the Société Française d'Informatique de Laboratoire (SFIL). The "Jeu de valeurs LOINC" is published once every six months. It is aligned with the "Nomenclature des Actes de Biologie Médicale (NABM)" since 2014. Its use is required in particular for:

- Producing and using medical laboratory test reports organised in accordance with the specifications of the "Medical laboratory test report" section of the "Cadre d'Interopérabilité des Systèmes d'Information de Santé (CI-SIS),
- guaranteeing the compatibility of these results and observations, when they come from different medical laboratories.

Unfortunately, as of now, medical laboratories use their own local terminologies to organise the biological data they produce [12]. This situation therefore leads to a growing need for a direct mapping between local terminologies and the standardised LOINC terminology [14,15]. Semi-automatic approaches and tools, including the one distributed by Regenstrief, are proposed to assist domain experts [9], but the mapping of local terminologies with LOINC remains time-consuming and requires a lot of human expertise [8]. With the exponential advances in automatic language processing driven by increasingly efficient artificial intelligence algorithms, our study aims at proposing an innovative solution to the problem of mapping these local terminologies with the LOINC encoding. To this end, our approach is designed by a multidisciplinary team of researchers in medicine, biology and artificial intelligence.

1.1 LOINC: A Closer Look

The LOINC terminology is a list of concepts referenced by a unique identifier, defining (1) analyses results for medical biology examinations, as well as (2) clinical and biometric observations included in the prescriptions for biology examinations. Each LOINC concept comprises a "long label" and a unique identification code. Each long label is composed of seven parts, (component, magnitude, etc.) separated into columns. LOINC is a pre-coordinated terminology that specifies only those combinations of atomic concepts that are allowed. For example, the six-part combination "Cortisol", "Moles/Volume", "Ponctuel", "Sérum/Plasma", "Numérique" and "Immunoanalyse" is relevant for the diagnosis of Cushing's syndrome and Addison's disease and has thus been integrated into LOINC with a code (83090-1). For improved coverage and completeness, it is possible to include additional concepts (post-coordination) into LOINC. In particular, users or developers can suggest new combinations of atomic concepts (proposed LOINC concepts) to the organisations in charge of LOINC maintenance.

1.2 Related Work

Existing approaches for mapping local terminologies with LOINC rely on extensive pre-processing of local terminologies to facilitate automated matching processing. Common pre-processing steps include harmonization of local terminologies [3], adoption of synonyms [6], resolution of abbreviations associated with an augmentation of local terms with definitions and annotations. Existing tools for mapping pre-processed local terminologies with LOINC typically compute concept similarities using the fully specified names. Using the example given above (LOINC code 83090-1), these names would be: "Cortisol", "Moles/Volume", "Ponctuel", "Sérum/Plasma", "Numérique" and "Immunoanalyse". Many of these studies use the Regenstrief LOINC Mapping Assistant (RELMA), which applies such a full name alignment strategy, based on exact and restrictive name matching [17]. Few studies have applied a linguistic alignment where a match can also be identified even for similar but slightly different concept names. Let us note, in particular, that such a full-name alignment strategy is linguistically dependant on the language in which the LOINC is written (i.e. English) Our approach, based on existing artificial intelligence techniques [7] combines both: (1) extensive pre-processing of local terminologies, (2) linguistic mapping using semantic similarity and (3) a structural mapping strategy by decomposing the local terminology into atomic concepts. It differs from other approaches by its use of linguistic processing techniques from the field of artificial intelligence. In the following, we will present our study followed by comparative results with the existing RELMA tool, revealing thereby the importance of taking linguistic considerations into the overall mapping stragegy.

2   Objective

In the interest of enhancing interoperability between French medical laboratory terminologies, we develop a linguistic algorithm for mapping these terminologies with "Jeu de valeurs LOINC", which is a French terminology based on LOINC (Logical Observation Identifiers Names and Codes). This paper presents a pilot case study with data obtained from the Biochemistry laboratory at the University Hospital of Montpellier, Hôpital Lapeyronie. The purpose of this study is to analyse the impact of using linguistic techniques to increase mapping quality and reduce cognitive and manual effort.

To address the linguistic complexities inherent to this task, we adopt a natural language processing (NLP) methodology. This allows us to (1) identify the linguistic factors that contribute to the mapping process, (2) develop a linguistically-enhanced, unified database of LOINC data combining French and international LOINC terminologies with additional UMLS concepts, (3) define a mapping strategy that exploits this database with state-of-the-art text-indexing techniques and (4) evaluate our algorithm by comparing it with the official mapping assistant RELMA in our pilot case study.

3   Materials and Methods

There are several challenges inherent in developing a linguistically-aware algorithm for mapping local terminologies with LOINC:

1. How does one approach the problem of multilingual mapping?

2. How does one handle cases where atomic concepts from LOINC are represented by their synonyms in the local terminologies?
3. How does one account for the structural discrepancies between the local terminologies and LOINC?

To address each of these challenges, we adopt a computational linguistic methodology which has been used in salient linguistic processing approaches in the field of artificial intelligence [REFERENCES]. In accordance with this methodology we proceed as follows:

Step 1: Linguistic and structural analysis of the input data
Step 2: Identification of linguistic markers that will facilitate mapping with LOINC
Step 3: Using these markers to define a semantically enriched LOINC knowledge base
Step 4: Develop a mapping strategy based on structural and linguistic processing of local terminologies.

We evaluate our approach on data obtained from the biochemistry laboratory of the CHU of Montpellier.

The rest of this section is devoted to detailing each of these steps individually.

3.1 Input Data: Structural and Linguistic Analyses

Following the afore-mentioned automatic mapping methodology, we first proceed with a fine-grained linguistic and structural analysis of the input data, in order to identify the elements that will serve as key points in the development of our mapping algorithm. We now present some of the results of our analyses; those that would fail when applying a full-name mapping strategy:

- Local terminology contains atomic concepts that need to be broken down into two different LOINC concepts (e.g. "Albumine plasmatique" becomes LOINC "composant" *Albumine* + LOINC "milieu" *Serum/Plasma*).
- Local terminology describes units such as *g/mol* while LOINC describes these as "grandeur" such as *Masse/Volume*.
- Local terminologies describe atomic concepts under a synonym of those used by the LOINC.
- Local terminology describes ratios using the word 'Ratio' (e.g. Ratio Sodium Créatinine) while these are represented using the symbol '/' in LOINC (e.g. Sodium/Creatinine).

3.2 Linguistic Markers: The Contributing Factor in the Mapping Process

The results of the linguistic and structural analyses allow us to define useful linguistic markers for the development of the final mapping algorithm. These markers are defined in the form of a list of linguistic rules that will be systematically applied to the whole dataset, in a pre-processing phase. For example, the adjective "fluoré (fluorinated)" in the local terminology is a linguistic marker that maps the input data with the atomic concept "Serum/Plasma" in LOINC. The identification of these linguistic markers is an essential step in the automatic mapping of the data because they allow the expert to avoid a manual step of defining correspondences as requested by the RELMA tool. It remains to be evaluated to what extent these linguistic markers are applicable to data sets from other laboratories.

3.3   Enriched Linguistic Model for Mapping LOINC Data

The official LOINC terminology is organised in a multi-column table, accessible in an Excel-type spreadsheet. The order of the entries does not reflect any structural organisation of the concepts, making it impossible to browse the data quickly. In order to overcome this difficulty, we develop an "enriched" LOINC database for our mapping algorithm. This database is defined using advanced data management technology, allowing:

- Hierarchical structuring of data,
- powerful text indexing for rapid identification of any keyword in the database, despite structural complexity.

Thanks to the functionalities provided by this technology, we were able to define the LOINC atomic concept pertaining to a "component" in a more refined way:
Component = [name] + follwing properties:

1. Analyte,
2. primary class,
3. synonyms,
4. semantic type,
5. syntactic type (ratio, challenge, etc.).

3.4   Mapping Strategy

The final step in the development of our LOINC mapping algorithm is to combine the previous steps into a mapping strategy. The strategy optimises the use of (1) our prior analyses and (2) our semantically enriched LOINC knowledge base and is as follows:

1. Identification of relevant columns in the input data,
2. prepossessing the data with the expert rules identified during the linguistic and structural analysis,
3. mapping in stages (multi-part matching) by addressing atomic concepts individually,
4. return the top 20 LOINC candidates for each input entry

4   Evaluation

Our approach has been evaluated as a proof of concept in a pilot study at the Lapeyronie University Hospital of Montpellier. Our results are promising and reflect the necessity of using a linguistic approach for mapping.

However, we note that the results presented in this section do not suffice for evaluating our apporoach, as they do not represent a representative sample of data.

4.1   Experimental Setup

We evaluate our approach by comparing our performance with that of the official LOINC mapping assistant RELMA, based on a gold-standard provided by our medical experts.

The local terminology contains 792 distinct entries. The gold-standard mapping between this local terminology and LOINC was established manually by two independent medical experts, both familiar with the laboratory nomenclature. The accuracy and consistency of inter-annotator mapping was manually ensured in case of discrepancies: the two experts were invited to discuss jointly to decide on a consensus for the disputed cases.

4.2   Results

Of the 792 entries contained in the input dataset, 86 (10.85%) were unmappable because they were incomplete or incompatible with LOINC. 706 entries were therefore processed by our mapping algorithm. We present our results with respect to the gold standard in Table 1.

Table 1. Mapping algorithm: results.

Total distinct entries	792
Total incomplete/inconsistent entries	86 (10.9%)
Total mapped entries	706 (89.1%)
Correctly mapped entries	593 (84%)
Unmapped entries	113 (16%)

Among the correct alignments proposed by our solution, 271 were processed by the RELMA tool officially proposed with the LOINC. Our comparative results are summarised in Table 2. Of the top 20 codes provided by each tool, the correct alignment code was contained in 100% of our results and 50.8% of those of RELMA.

Semi-automatic mapping times were also measured, with all 792 entries processed in 4 h and 40 min by a medical expert, i.e. 170 entries mapped per hour.

Table 2. Mapping algorithm vs RELMA.

	Our algorithm	RELMA
Mapped entries	271	271
Correctly mapped	271 (100%)	138 (50.9%)
Incorrectly mapped	0	133 (49.1%)

Although few studies mention local terminology mapping times with LOINC, we can compare this time with that achieved during an evaluation of RELMA by a German team, which found an average of 60 entries mapped per hour [17]. Our system is thus 2.8 times faster than RELMA.

4.3   Discussion

The heterogeneity of field data and the often long history with which laboratory databases have been designed and maintained, imposes an effort to pre-process the data even before applying algorithms to align the data with the LOINC repository. This pre-processing step can only be effective if the data owner has a good understanding of the LOINC nomenclature data structure and what types of relevant information are to be considered in their own data, to ensure the best performance of the automatic alignment. This work requires training time for the domain expert medical biologists involved [4]. The question of the interoperability of LOINC-coded data deserves to be asked concerning LOINC codes relating to measurements for which the technique is not specified, even though it constitutes a specificity to be taken into consideration for the correct interpretation of the associated biological result. One example is "creatinine", for which it is recommended in France to use an "enzymatic" (as opposed to "colorimetric") technique to estimate the glomerular filtration rate according to the CKD-EPI equation [13]. Thus two laboratories measuring creatinine in serum and expressed in moles/volume, but where one laboratory uses an enzymatic assay and the other a colorimetric assay, would share the same LOINC code, raising the question of the comparability of the result for the same patient visiting each of these two laboratories. Thus, other teams have suggested the need to associate additional information with the LOINC format in order to correctly interpret the associated biological result [2] This additional information relates to the characteristics of the analyser (technique, reagent) or to specific comments on the result that should be communicated in relation to the test results. All coding systems have weaknesses and, in particular, the "uncoded" system (currently used in France) of using highly ambiguous and interchangeable names for tests also has weaknesses. Thus, despite these limitations, we believe that the structuring of biological data according to the LOINC reference system has the merit of giving medical laboratories a structuring framework, which will enable them to make better secondary use of the data they produce. Based on our positive results, which are satisfactory for the expert biologists who use it, we propose to make sustained efforts to support medical laboratories in the correct use of this data format. These efforts must involve: experts in the field (hospital and private medical biologists), government agencies such as the Agence du Numérique en Santé, and digital health manufacturers. The latter can facilitate the adoption of this format by proposing solutions for automatic transcoding of field data.

5   Conclusion

This paper presents a pilot case study evaluated upon data obtained from the Biochemistry laboratory at the University Hospital of Montpellier, Hôpital Lapeyronie. We analyse the impact of using linguistic techniques to increase mapping quality and reduce cognitive and manual effort.

Our pilot case study shows that computational assistance in aligning terminologies makes it 3 times faster for domain experts. The significant difference in performance between RELMA and our tool reflects the impact of addressing the linguistic challenges involved in the mapping process. RELMA, developed for the English language, drops significantly in performance levels when compared with a mapping algorithm tailored to the French language.

References

1. Amith, M.F., He, Z., Bian, J., Lossio-Ventura, J.A., Tao, C.: Assessing the practice of biomedical ontology evaluation: gaps and opportunities. J. Biomed. Inform. **80**, 1–13 (2018). https://doi.org/10.1016/j.jbi.2018.02.010, https://www.ncbi.nlm.nih. gov/pmc/articles/PMC5882531/
2. Drenkhahna, C.: The LOINC content model and its limitations of usage in the laboratory domain. In: Digital Personalized Health and Medicine, p. 6 (2020)
3. Fidahussein, M., Vreeman, D.J.: A corpus-based approach for automated LOINC mapping. J. Am. Med. Inform. Assoc. **21**(1), 64–72 (2014). https://doi. org/10.1136/amiajnl-2012-001159, https://www.ncbi.nlm.nih.gov/pmc/articles/ PMC3912728/
4. Fiebeck, J., et al.: Implementing LOINC - current status and ongoing work at a Medical University, p. 7 (2019)
5. Gkoutos, G.V., Schofield, P.N., Hoehndorf, R.: The anatomy of phenotype ontologies: principles, properties and applications. Briefi. Bioinform. **19**(5), 1008–1021 (2017). https://doi.org/10.1093/bib/bbx035, https://www.ncbi.nlm.nih.gov/pmc/ articles/PMC6169674/
6. Jung, B.K., et al..: Report on the Project for Establishment of the standardized Korean laboratory terminology database, 2015. J. Korean Med. Sci. **32**(4), 695–699 (2017). https://doi.org/10.3346/jkms.2017.32.4.695, https://www.ncbi. nlm.nih.gov/pmc/articles/PMC5334171/
7. Kaci, S., Patel, N., Prince, V.: From NL preference expressions to comparative preference statements: a preliminary study in eliciting preferences for customised decision support. In: 2014 IEEE 26th International Conference on Tools with Artificial Intelligence, pp. 591–598. IEEE (2014)

8. Kim, H., El-Kareh, R., Goel, A., Vineet, F., Chapman, W.W.: An approach to improve LOINC mapping through augmentation of local test names. J. Biomed. Inform. **45**(4), 651–657 (2012). https://doi.org/10.1016/j.jbi.2011.12.004, https://www.ncbi.nlm.nih.gov/pmc/articles/PMC3340474/

9. Kopanitsa, G.: Application of a regenstrief RELMA vol 6.6 to map Russian laboratory terms to LOINC. Methods Inf. Med. **55**(02), 177–181 (2016). https://doi.org/10.3414/ME15-01-0068, http://www.thieme-connect.de/DOI/DOI?10.3414/ME15-01-0068

10. McDonald, C.J., et al.: LOINC, a universal standard for identifying laboratory observations: a 5-year update. Clin. Chem. **49**(4), 624–633 (2003). https://doi.org/10.1373/49.4.624

11. Poli, R., Healy, M., Kameas, A. (eds.): Theory and Applications of Ontology: Computer Applications. Springer, Netherlands (2010). https://doi.org/10.1007/978-90-481-8847-5, https://www.springer.com/gp/book/9789048188468

12. Rosenbloom, S.T., Miller, R.A., Johnson, K.B., Elkin, P.L., Brown, S.H.: Interface terminologies: facilitating direct entry of clinical data into electronic health record systems. J. Am. Med. Inform. Assoc. **13**(3), 277–288 (2006). https://doi.org/10.1197/jamia.M1957, https://www.ncbi.nlm.nih.gov/pmc/articles/PMC1513664/

13. de Santé, H.A.: Évaluation du débit de filtration glomérulaire et du dosage de la créatininémie dans le diagnostic de la maladie rénale chronique chez l'adulte. Biotribune Mag. **41**(1), 6–9 (2011). https://doi.org/10.1007/s11834-011-0067-3, http://link.springer.com/10.1007/s11834-011-0067-3

14. Uchegbu, C., Jing, X.: The potential adoption benefits and challenges of LOINC codes in a laboratory department: a case study. Health Inf. Sci. Syst. **5**(1) (2017). https://doi.org/10.1007/s13755-017-0027-8, https://www.ncbi.nlm.nih.gov/pmc/articles/PMC5636728/

15. Wade, G., Rosenbloom, S.T.: Experiences mapping a legacy interface terminology to SNOMED CT. BMC Med. Inf. Decision Making **8**(Suppl 1), S3 (2008). https://doi.org/10.1186/1472-6947-8-S1-S3, https://www.ncbi.nlm.nih.gov/pmc/articles/PMC2582790/

16. Wang, K.C.: Standard lexicons, coding systems and ontologies for interoperability and semantic computation in imaging. J. Digit. Imag. **31**(3), 353–360 (2018). https://doi.org/10.1007/s10278-018-0069-8, http://link.springer.com/10.1007/s10278-018-0069-8

17. Zunner, C., Bürkle, T., Prokosch, H.U., Ganslandt, T.: Mapping local laboratory interface terms to LOINC at a German university hospital using RELMA V.5: a semi-automated approach. J. Am. Med. Inform. Assoc. **20**(2), 293–297 (2013). https://doi.org/10.1136/amiajnl-2012-001063, https://academic.oup.com/jamia/article-lookup/doi/10.1136/amiajnl-2012-001063

Volunteer Computing Project SiDock@home for Virtual Drug Screening Against SARS-CoV-2

Natalia Nikitina[1]($^{(\boxtimes)}$) (iD), Maxim Manzyuk[2] (iD), Črtomir Podlipnik[3] (iD), and Marko Jukić[4,5]($^{(\boxtimes)}$) (iD)

[1] Karelian Research Center of the Russian Academy of Sciences,
Institute of Applied Mathematical Research, 185910 Petrozavodsk, Russia
nikitina@krc.karelia.ru
[2] Internet Portal BOINC.Ru, Moscow, Russia
[3] Faculty of Chemistry and Chemical Technology,
University of Ljubljana, 1000 Ljubljana, Slovenia
[4] Laboratory of Physical Chemistry and Chemical Thermodynamics, Faculty of Chemistry and Chemical Engineering, University of Maribor, 2000 Maribor, Slovenia
[5] Faculty of Mathematics, Natural Sciences and Information Technologies,
University of Primorska, 6000 Koper, Slovenia

Abstract. In this paper, we describe a volunteer computing project SiDock@home aimed at high-throughput virtual screening of a specially developed library of small compounds against a set of targets playing important roles in the life-cycle of the virus. The originality of the screening library and the molecular docking software allows us to obtain new knowledge about chemical space in relation to SARS-CoV-2. At the same time, the existing volunteer computing community provides us with a large computational power. Having risen to a size of a modern supercomputer in several months, SiDock@home becomes an independent general drug discovery project, with its first mission targeting SARS-CoV-2.

Keywords: Distributed computing · Volunteer computing · BOINC · Desktop grid · Virtual screening · Molecular docking · SARS-CoV-2

1 Introduction

Since the very early stages of COVID-19 pandemic onset, scientists all over the world have employed different high-performance computing (HPC) systems to

Supported by the Scholarship of the President of the Russian Federation for young scientists and graduate students (project SP-609.2021.5), the Slovenian Ministry of Science and Education infrastructure, project grant HPC-RIVR, by the Slovenian Research Agency (ARRS), programme P2-0046 and J1-2471, the Physical Chemistry programme grant P1-0201; Slovenian Ministry of Education, Science and Sports programme grant OP20.04342.

© IFIP International Federation for Information Processing 2021
Published by Springer Nature Switzerland AG 2021
A. Byrski et al. (Eds.): ANTICOVID 2021, IFIP AICT 616, pp. 23–34, 2021.
https://doi.org/10.1007/978-3-030-86582-5_3

fight against SARS-CoV-2; see, e.g., [4] for a regularly updated detailed overview. There are nationwide and cross-nation research initiatives that provide scientists with HPC resources such as rojects supported by the world's leading supercomputer Fugaku (Japan) [23], the COVID-19 High-Performance Computing Consortium (USA) [25], the Exscalate4CoV project (EU) [12] and many others.

Apart from traditional HPC systems, there are alternative capabilities such as Desktop Grids that combine non-dedicated geographically distributed computing resources (typically, desktop computers) connected to the central server by the Internet or a local access network and performing computations for the Desktop Grid in their idle time. The resources are provided by the volunteer community or by individuals and organisations related to the performed research.

Desktop Grids hold a special place among the HPC systems due to their enormous potential and, at the same time, high availability to teams of any size, even at the very early stages of research.

Today, the potential of Desktop Grids is estimated as hundreds of exaflops [1]. It is much more than the total power of all existing supercomputers. In particular, a volunteer computing project Folding@home gathered the resources of more than an exaflops in early 2020 and became the first world's exascale system, more powerful than the top 100 supercomputers altogether [10].

Like most citizen science initiatives, BOINC projects on bio-medicine have always attracted many volunteer participants due to their socially important subjects. With the onset of a pandemic, the number of participants raised as well as the number of projects. In this paper, we try to review the BOINC projects targeting the coronavirus and present a new project named SiDock@home aimed at drug discovery and its first mission: the fight against SARS-CoV-2.

The paper has the following structure. In Sect. 2, we overview the current state of the BOINC middleware for organising Desktop Grids. We also describe existing BOINC-based projects targeting SARS-CoV-2. In Sect. 3, we describe the BOINC-based volunteer computing project named SiDock@home. In Sect. 4, we conclude the paper and provide plans for the project's future.

2   BOINC-Based Projects Targeting SARS-CoV-2

2.1   BOINC Middleware

To organise and manage Desktop Grid-based distributed computations, a number of software platforms are used. The most popular platform among them is BOINC (Berkeley Open Infrastructure for Desktop Computing) [1]. Among the 157 active largest projects on volunteer computing, 89 are based on BOINC [9]; that is, BOINC can be considered a *de-facto* standard for the operation of volunteer computing projects. The platform is an actively developing Open Source software and provides rich functionality.

BOINC has a server-client architecture. The server generates a large number of tasks that are mutually independent parts of a computationally intensive problem. When a client computer is idle, it requests work from the server, receives tasks, and independently processes them. Upon finishing, it reports results back to the server. The results are then stored in the database for further usage.

Such an architecture has proven to be efficient and highly scalable for solving computationally-intensive problems of the bag-of-tasks type. The total average performance of active BOINC-based research projects is estimated as 28.5 petaflops/s [3] using an internal benchmark averaged by the last 90 days.

Due to the different benchmarks, specifics of the solved computationally-intensive problems and particular features of computing systems, it is complicated to compare the performance of BOINC-based Desktop Grids with supercomputers. Nevertheless, there exist various techniques to estimate the scale of Desktop Grids. E.g., in [22], we show that a volunteer computing project develops to the scale of a modern supercomputer in the first months of its operation (see Table 1). During periods of high workload (such as community competitions among BOINC teams), performance of a Desktop Grid increases several-fold.

Table 1. Available computational resources of the project SiDock@home during the testing phase and the main phase (in bold), as of March 23, 2021.

Average performance, teraflops/s	Peak performance, teraflops/s	Average load, active threads	Registered computers	Registered participants
23 (**115**)	35 (**216**)	1180 (**5895**)	934 (**9193**)	272 (**2402**)

The urgency of the SARS-CoV-2-related research has also impacted a new computational model stemming from BOINC, Science United [28]. In this model, participants specify subject areas they wish to contribute to instead of concrete projects. The administration can allocate more CPU/GPU power to priority problems, such as fighting SARS-CoV-2 [29]. Today, the combined account of Science United takes first place by daily credit [3], provided by 5 386 computers. A significant part of this capacity is performing SARS-CoV-2-related projects.

2.2 BOINC Projects

For decades, the volunteer computing community has provided researchers with many computational resources ready at hand. It contributed to the development of various theoretical and empirical methods. The gained experience allowed several research groups to obtain first results at the very early stages of the fight against coronavirus. Let us overview existing public BOINC-based projects targeting SARS-CoV-2, their aims and recent results.

Rosetta@home project performs computer modelling of the end state of the folded proteins [14]. The previous experience and available volunteer resources allowed the scientific team to accurately predict the structure of the key SARS-CoV-2 spike protein (key role in pathogenesis) several weeks before its description by cryo-electron microscopy [37]. A series of previous results became a basis for *de novo* design of picomolar SARS-CoV-2 mini protein inhibitors [5].

World Community Grid, a large-scale umbrella project [36], launched the sub-project OpenPandemics [24] in May 2020 as a platform for a quick start of research in case of any pandemic. At its current mission, OpenPandemics targets the search for potential inhibitors of various SARS-CoV-2 proteins using virtual screening of large libraries of chemical compounds.

TN-Grid project [33], in its sub-project gene@home, explores human gene regulatory networks for receptor proteins of SARS-CoV-2 and other viruses. To date, results include the expansion of the networks of genes associated with two non-viral diseases, identification of 22 and 36 genes to be evaluated as novel targets for already approved drugs [2].

IberCIVIS, another long-running umbrella project [13], has run the sub-project COVID-Phym aimed at the virtual screening of existing drugs for SARS-CoV-2 targets to find compounds able to block the replication mechanism of the coronavirus. The performed molecular docking allowed to deeper investigate the reasons why remdesivir and tenofovir had shown only partial evidence of improving clinical outcomes in clinical trials and observational studies [8]. The results may lay in the basis for the development of tenofovir-based drug complexes.

BOINC@TACC project hosted a large part of jobs of the virtual screening held by the University of Texas [34]. The research aimed at developing the molecular structure of a protease inhibitor that would target the coronavirus.

In Fig. 1(a), we illustrate the performance of the active BOINC projects in teraflops/s. One observes that more than 75% of the total performance is contributed by GPU-based applications, which currently do not include SARS-CoV-2 related research (as of April 2021). The latter projects constitute only 3.6% of the total performance of BOINC.

However, as shown in Fig. 1(b), breakdown by the number of active computers is the opposite. Note that a computer can participate in multiple BOINC projects, but detailed statistics on each computer are not available. For this reason, we do not chart intersections. Still, the data shows that SARS-CoV-2 related projects are run by between 40% and 75% of computers participating in BOINC. The data on active participants (Table 2) supports this rough estimate.

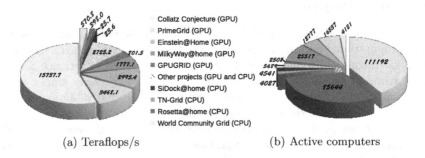

(a) Teraflops/s   (b) Active computers

Fig. 1. Comparative performance of the active BOINC projects: Top-5 (in gray), performing SARS-CoV-2-related research (in color), and others (dashed).

Table 2. The number of active participants, as of April 5, 2021.

All BOINC projects excl. ASIC	World Community Grid	Rosetta@home	SiDock@home	TN-Grid
79 071	37 062 (47%)	30 552 (37%)	1 620 (2%)	750 (0.9%)

To summarise, existing public SARS-CoV-2-related BOINC projects base on moderately CPU-intensive applications and attract thousands of participants. Meanwhile, the BOINC community provides a large number of GPU resources that may boost a research project.

In the next section, we describe a BOINC-based research project named *SiDock@home*, created and supported by our team, aimed at drug discovery, with the first mission of fighting SARS-CoV-2.

3   SiDock@home Project

3.1   Setup of a BOINC Project

In March 2020, a Slovenian research group led by Dr. Črtomir Podlipnik and Dr. Marko Jukić initiated a citizen science project *"Citizen science and the fight against the coronavirus"* (COVID.SI) [11] in the field of drug design and medicinal chemistry. The project is aimed at drug discovery, and first of all, against coronavirus infection, using high-throughput virtual screening (HTVS) [16,31]. To achieve the goal, the authors performed molecular docking using a library of ten million of small molecules against multiple potential therapeutic targets.

The design of the HTVS problem allows to scale it according to the needs of researchers easily. However, even with an optimal computational process organisation, the throughput is always limited by the properties of available high-performance computing resources.

Upon the first successful results, the need for extension of the computational capacity became apparent. To complement and scale the available computational resources, we created a new SiDock@home, the BOINC-based extension of COVID.SI. The project was announced to the community in October 2020. As we have noted above, the volunteer contributions summed up to a scale of a modern supercomputer during the first five months, and SiDock@home organically grew into a sizable, independent and competent research project for general drug design. We provide the performance dynamics in more detail in [22].

The project SiDock@home [32] was created based on the BOINC middleware. The project's server part was deployed in an Ubuntu 18.04 LTS-based machine under system configuration of 2 Xeon 6140 cores, 8 Gb RAM, 32 Gb SSD and 512 Gb HDD. At the client's part, the project supports Windows, Linux and MacOS 64-bit operating systems, including Linux on ARM (Raspberry Pi).

3.2 High-Throughput Virtual Screening in SiDock@home

Targets. Following the course of research of COVID.SI, we considered a set of 59 targets to screen first of all (see Table 3). 3D structural models of the targets were generated by the D-I-TASSER/C-I-TASSER pipeline [19].

We started virtual screening from 3CL^{pro}, the main viral protease, a valuable therapeutic target that possesses no mutations in the pandemically relevant variants such as such as B.1.1.7, B.1.351, P.1 and B.1.617. A small library of chemical compounds available to order had been already screened prior to the start of SiDock@home [17]. The study of a larger library may help to extend the structural knowledge about the target an improve the prioritisation of compounds for ordering and testing in a laboratory.

Another essential viral protease, PL^{pro}, regulating SARS-CoV-2 viral spread and innate immunity [30], was studied with two different catalytic active sites.

The next target, RdRp, is frequently used in research studies as a potential target to inhibit viral replication. Specifically, it is SARS-CoV-2 RNA-dependent RNA polymerase, an enzyme which coronavirus SARS-CoV-2 uses for the replication of its genome and the transcription of its genes.

Currently, the project is screening the library against the envelope (E) protein that is known to form a pore spanning the lipid bilayer membrane of the virus [18]. The research suggests that inhibition of the E protein viroporin could limit pathogenicity and could be of therapeutic value.

Each target corresponds to a separate computational experiment, and the next experiment's setup may depend on the results of the previous ones. If necessary, one may perform several computational experiments in parallel.

It is observed [15] that in Desktop Grids, the final part of a computational experiment may take much time to complete due to the unreliable character of the computational system. To decrease the runtime and obtain the complete picture on a considered target, we applied such a technical method as decreasing the task deadline. In BOINC, if a task does not finish upon the deadline, it is considered lost, and the server issues another replica of the task.

There is another possibility to speed up the completion of a target by announcing a competition in the BOINC community. The experience shows [22] that the performance of the project increases several-fold in such periods.

Ligands. To prepare the library of small compounds, we conglomerated multiple commercial and academic sources of 2D molecular structures, cleaned the structures, checked for errors, ionised and calculated 3D structures using the algorithms partly described in [26,35]. The resulting library contains about 1 000 000 000 compounds readily available for molecular docking software.

The relatively small size of a separate compound and the corresponding task allow graining the computational problem of HTVS as desired. In the case of a BOINC-based Desktop Grid, the common practice is to divide the problem into the tasks that run on an average desktop computer for the order of hours.

BOINC middleware allows running native applications without changing their source code using the wrapper program [38]. We used this mechanism to bring molecular docking software RxDock [20,27] to the Desktop Grid.

Table 3. Targets for the first set of computational experiments in SiDock@home.

Target ID	The protein	Organism	Source of structure	PDB code
1–21	3CL^{pro}	SARS-2	Snapshots from MD trajectory	
26–34	Spike Protein	SARS/MERS/ SARS-2	Crystalographic structures	2AJF, 2DD8, 3SCL, 5X58, 6ACK, 6LZG, 6M0J, 6M17, 6VW1
35–37	DHODH	Human	Crystalographic structures	4IGH, 4JTU, 4OQV
41–48	PL Pro	SARS/MERS/ SARS-2	Crystalographic structures	2FE8, 3MP2, 4OW0, 6W9C, 6WRH, 6WUU, 6WX4, 6WZU
49–50	FURIN	Human	Crystalographic structures	5JXH, 5MIM
51–54	Methyl Transferase	SARS-2	Crystalographic structures	6W4H, 6W61, 7C2I, 7C2J
55–56	E Protein	SARS/SARS-2	NMR/Homology model	5X29 (SARS) 5X29 Homology (SARS-2)
58–59	PL^{pro}	SARS-2	Homology models	Based on 3E9S, 5E6J, 6W9C

Following the first molecular docking results, we divided the small molecules library into packages of 2 000 entries. The tasks of such size take about one-two hours to complete on an average desktop computer. However, the runtimes for different targets may vary significantly. The project's workflow is not bound to the fixed package size and supports any other static or dynamic library division.

HTVS Protocol. To reduce the computational time several-fold, we implemented a simple multi-step protocol according to [21] rather than docking the entire library in exhaustive mode. Algorithm 1 describes the workflow for a set of N ligands. Here, the values M (the maximal number of runs), R_1 (the number of runs to decide if a ligand shows a binding score better than S_1 and thus passes to the second stage), R_2 (the number of runs to decide if a ligand shows a binding score better than S_2 and thus passes to the third stage) are pre-determined using the utility `rbhtfinder` to optimise the HTVS process for a given library.

HTVS Setup. BOINC provides several mechanisms to increase the effective performance of a Desktop Grid despite unreliable computational nodes.

At the moment, we have addressed two main problems that impact the efficiency of the HTVS: overdue tasks that may significantly slow down an experiment and erroneous results that cause "false-negative" outcomes. To overcome

Algorithm 1. An HTVS protocol for N ligands and a maximum of M runs

---

 1: **for** $ligand = 1, 2, \ldots, N$ **do**
 2:     **for** $run = 1, 2, \ldots, R_1$ **do**   ▷ First stage
 3:         Run molecular docking for $ligand$ and save the best $score$ and $pose$
 4:         **if** $score \geq S_1$ **then go to 13**
 5:     **end for**
 6:     **for** $run = R_1 + 1, R_1 + 2, \ldots, R_2$ **do**   ▷ Second stage
 7:         Run molecular docking for $ligand$ and save the best $score$ and $pose$
 8:         **if** $score \geq S_2$ **then go to 13**
 9:     **end for**
10:     **for** $run = R_2 + 1, R_2 + 2, \ldots, M$ **do**   ▷ Third stage
11:         Run molecular docking for $ligand$ and save the best $score$ and $pose$
12:     **end for**
13:     Output the best $score$ and $pose$ for $ligand$
14: **end for**

---

the first problem, we set a relatively short deadline of 72 h. To overcome the second one, we set a quorum of two and implemented a result validation algorithm that checks if the log files show equal non-empty sets of ligands having been processed. The initial replication level is two instances of a task that are always sent to different users and hosts to enable cross-checking.

Thus, a task's input data contains a package of $N = 2\,000$ small molecules, the target files and the description of an HTVS protocol. Output data contains the docking results and the docking log. The latter is used to validate the results automatically and achieve a quorum.

Molecular Docking Software. To perform molecular docking on the first target, we used Open Source software RxDock. At the same time, we employed an independent fork CmDock [7] by the COVID.SI team, aimed at the open-science approach, utilisation of graphics processing units (GPUs) and introduction of modern docking analysis tools and improved docking algorithms. For another two targets, we used the two docking applications in parallel. Later on, we completely switched to CmDock.

Results. The described setup allowed us to perform HTVS on the complete library for four targets in five months. The results include compounds readily available to purchase as well as synthesizable compounds, and are in line with the previously started research of the group.

After initial filtering by the predicted binding energies, the results are subject to calculation of physicochemical properties and clustering analysis. In Fig. 2, we illustrate the chemical diversity of the 5141 compounds that showed predicted binding energy at most –35.0 kcal/mol in the first experiment (target 3CLpro). Here, we set the energy threshold so as to proceed on a previous study [17].

The clustering analysis performed on calculated pairwise similarities revealed 711 clusters including 519 non-singleton ones with 0.807 merge distance, according to the Kelley criterion. Therefore, the results show good chemical diversity and comply well with conventional principles of HTVS.

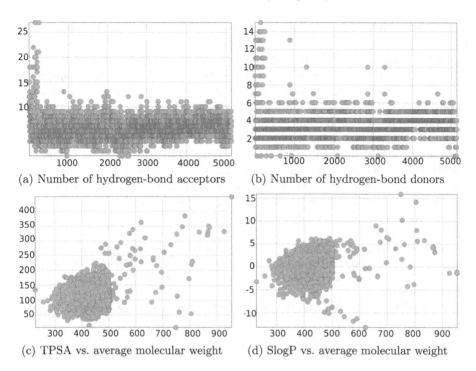

(a) Number of hydrogen-bond acceptors   (b) Number of hydrogen-bond donors

(c) TPSA vs. average molecular weight   (d) SlogP vs. average molecular weight

Fig. 2. Physicochemical properties of the set of selected 5141 compounds docked against target 3CLpro. Abbreviations used: TPSA – topological polar surface area; SlogP – logarithm of the enhanced atomic partition coefficient.

As of June 2021, we are post-processing the obtained results and performing HTVS for the fifth target in parallel. With hits obtained for several targets, we focus on viral proteases and are in the phase of obtaining physical samples of compounds for wet-lab testing. We are also working on SARS-CoV-2 spike protein (Sprot) and its mutations, investigating how they are connected to pathogenicity and how to design compounds on the system.

4   Conclusion

HPC systems have been widely employed to fight against SARS-CoV-2 since the very early stages of COVID-19 pandemic onset. Desktop Grid systems serve as an efficient, highly scalable tool to complement traditional HPC systems, with an estimated potential of hundreds of exaflops. In this paper, we overviewed the existing research projects operating on BOINC-based Desktop Grids and introduced another one, SiDock@home, created and supported by our team.

The project SiDock@home is aimed at drug discovery by performing an HTVS of the specially designed small molecules library. Its first and current mission is HTVS against a set of targets related to the life cycle of SARS-CoV-

2. However, SiDock@home is becoming an independent general drug discovery project. The project will eventually require large amounts of computational resources – and the BOINC community is ready to kindly provide them.

The future work is planned in several directions. Firstly, we plan to implement a GPU version of the application CmDock, which will dramatically increase the performance of the HTVS. Simultaneously, we need to increase the rate of results post-processing accordingly, most likely, in a distributed way.

Secondly, we will develop a more sophisticated HTVS protocol for optimising the computational time and hits discovery rate. Thirdly, we aim to extend the results and examine a "pan-coronavirus target", or, more specifically, a set of different coronavirus targets to design an inhibitor that works on multiple ones.

Finally, we will continue to future potential dangers such as targets on the SADS syndrome caused by an HKU2-related coronavirus.

Acknowledgements. The first initial library (one billion of compounds) was prepared with the generous help of Microsoft that donated computational resources in the Azure cloud platform [6]. We all from COVID.SI are grateful and looking forward to future collaborations.

We wholeheartedly thank all BOINC participants for their contributions.

References

1. Anderson, D.P.: BOINC: a platform for volunteer computing. J. Grid Comput. **18**(1), 99–122 (2020)
2. Blanzieri, E., et al.: A computing system for discovering causal relationships among human genes to improve drug repositioning. IEEE Trans. Emerg. Topics Comput. pp. 1–1 (2020). https://doi.org/10.1109/TETC.2020.3031024
3. BOINC combined - Detailed stats – BOINCstats/BAM! https://www.boincstats.com/stats/-5/project/detail. Accessed 30 Jun 2021
4. By Editorial Team: The history of supercomputing vs. COVID-19. https://www.hpcwire.com/2021/03/09/the-history-of-supercomputing-vs-covid-19. Accessed 18 Mar 2021
5. Cao, L., et al.: De novo design of picomolar SARS-CoV-2 miniprotein inhibitors. Science **370**(6515), 426–431 (2020). https://doi.org/10.1126/science.abd9909, https://science.sciencemag.org/content/370/6515/426
6. Cloud Computing Services – Microsoft Azure. https://azure.microsoft.com/en-us/. Accessed 30 Jun 2021
7. CmDock. https://gitlab.com/Jukic/cmdock. Accessed 30 Jun 2021
8. De Salazar, P.M., Ramos, J., Cruz, V.L., Polo, R., Del Amo, J., Martínez-Salazar, J.: Tenofovir and remdesivir ensemble docking with the SARS-CoV-2 polymerase and template-nascent RNA. Authorea Preprints (2020)
9. Distributed Computing - Computing Platforms. http://distributedcomputing.info/platforms.html. Accessed 30 Jun 2021
10. Folding@home - fighting disease with a world wide distributed super computer. https://foldingathome.org. Accessed 30 Jun 2021
11. Home - COVID.SI. https://covid.si/en. Accessed 30 Jun 2021
12. Home [Exscalate4COV consortium]. https://www.exscalate4cov.eu/index.html. Accessed 30 Jun 2021

13. IberCIVIS. https://boinc.ibercivis.es/. Accessed 30 Jun 2021
14. Institute for Protein design, University of Washington: Rosetta's role in fighting coronavirus. https://www.ipd.uw.edu/2020/02/rosettas-role-in-fighting-coronavirus. Accessed 30 Jun 2021
15. Ivashko, E., Nikitina, N.: Replication of "tail" computations in a desktop grid project. In: Voevodin, V., Sobolev, S. (eds.) RuSCDays 2020. CCIS, vol. 1331, pp. 611–621. Springer, Cham (2020). https://doi.org/10.1007/978-3-030-64616-5_52
16. Jukič, M., Janežič, D., Bren, U.: Ensemble docking coupled to linear interaction energy calculations for identification of coronavirus main protease (3CLpro) noncovalent small-molecule inhibitors. Molecules **25**(24), 5808 (2020)
17. Jukič, M., Škrlj, B., Tomšič, G., Pleško, S., Podlipnik, Č, Bren, U.: Prioritisation of compounds for 3CLpro inhibitor development on SARS-CoV-2 variants. Molecules **26**(10), 3003 (2021)
18. Mandala, V.S., McKay, M.J., Shcherbakov, A.A., Dregni, A.J., Kolocouris, A., Hong, M.: Structure and drug binding of the SARS-CoV-2 envelope protein transmembrane domain in lipid bilayers. Nat. Struct. Mole. Biol. **27**(12), 1202–1208 (2020)
19. Modeling of the SARS-COV-2 Genome using I-TASSER. https://zhanglab.ccmb.med.umich.edu/COVID-19. Accessed 30 Jun 2021
20. Morley, S.D., Afshar, M.: Validation of an empirical RNA-ligand scoring function for fast flexible docking using RiboDock®. J. Comput.-aided Mole. Des. **18**(3), 189–208 (2004)
21. Multi-step protocol for HTVS – RxDock 0.1.0 documentation. https://www.rxdock.org/documentation/devel/html/user-guide/multi-step-protocol-for-htvs.html. Accessed 30 Jun 2021
22. Nikitina, N., Manzyuk, M., Podlipnik, C., Jukić, M.: Performance estimation of a BOINC-based Desktop Grid for large-scale molecular docking. In: 16th International Conference on Parallel Computing Technologies,PaCT-2021, submitted, 2021
23. Ongoing Projects – RIKEN Center for Computational Science RIKEN Website. https://www.r-ccs.riken.jp/en/fugaku/research/covid-19/projects. Accessed 30 Jun 2021
24. OpenPandemics - COVID-19 – Research – World Community Grid. https://www.worldcommunitygrid.org/research/opn1/overview.do. accessed 30 Jun 2021
25. Projects – COVID-19 HPC Consortium. https://covid19-hpc-consortium.org/projects. Accessed 30 Jun 2021
26. Puranen, J.S., Vainio, M.J., Johnson, M.S.: Accurate conformation-dependent molecular electrostatic potentials for high-throughput in silico drug discovery. J. Comput. Chem. **31**(8), 1722–1732 (2010)
27. Ruiz-Carmona, S., et al.: rDock: a fast, versatile and open source program for docking ligands to proteins and nucleic acids. PLoS Comput. Biol. **10**(4), e1003571 (2014)
28. Science United. https://scienceunited.org. Accessed 30 Jun 2021
29. Science United and COVID-19. https://scienceunited.org/forum_thread.php?id=132Accessed 30 Jun 2021
30. Shin, D., et al.: Papain-like protease regulates SARS-CoV-2 viral spread and innate immunity. Nature **587**(7835), 657–662 (2020)
31. Shoichet, B.K., McGovern, S.L., Wei, B., Irwin, J.J.: Lead discovery using molecular docking. Curr. Opin. Chem. Biol. **6**(4), 439–446 (2002)
32. SiDock@home. https://sidock.si/sidock Accessed 30 Jun 2021

33. TN-Grid. http://gene.disi.unitn.it/test/. Accessed 30 Jun 2021
34. UTEP school of pharmacy developing COVID-19 vaccine, drug treatments using supercomputing. https://www.utep.edu/newsfeed/campus/utep-school-of-pharmacy-developing-covid-19-vaccine,-drug-treatments-using-supercomputing.html (2021). Accessed 30 Jun 2021
35. Vainio, M.J., Johnson, M.S.: Generating conformer ensembles using a multiobjective genetic algorithm. J. Chem. Inf. Model. **47**(6), 2462–2474 (2007)
36. World Community Grid - home. https://www.worldcommunitygrid.org/. Accessed 30 Jun 2021
37. Wrapp, D., et al.: Cryo-EM structure of the 2019-nCoV spike in the prefusion conformation. Science **367**(6483), 1260–1263 (2020)
38. WrapperApp - BOINC. https://boinc.berkeley.edu/trac/wiki/WrapperApp. Accessed 30 Jun 2021

An Empirical Investigation of Pandemic Impact on IT Students' Educational Schedule

Natalia Shakhovska⬤, Ivanna Dronyuk⬤, Zoreslava Shpak⬤,
and Myroslava Klapchuk$^{(\boxtimes)}$⬤

Lviv Polytechnic National University, 12 S. Bandera Street, Lviv 79013, Ukraine
{ivanna.m.droniuk,myroslava.i.klapchuk}@lpnu.ua

Abstract. The novel coronavirus disease (COVID-19) forced the Ukrainian government to introduce lockdown on March 12, 2020. In addition, the transition to distance learning in schools and universities has posed new challenges to the entire education system and young people. In this study, a survey of IT students was conducted using Google forms. The questions in the questionnaire were aimed at studying the impact of online learning on the distribution of the students' day and the impact of the pandemic on the emotional state of a young person. The survey results showed significant changes in the daily schedule of students caused by the pandemic crisis. Thus, a remarkable increase in computer time can be a negative factor in influencing the health and emotional state of the younger generation.

Keywords: COVID-19 · University students · Online learning · Home education · Pandemics

1 Introduction

In 2020, humanity has entered a crisis period caused by a new user pandemic, called COVID-19. The study of the impact of pandemics on various areas of human life is just beginning. But it is safe to say that such a phenomenon in various areas of human activity will be long-term. In many cases, this effect is complicated to predict because of many factors that have never been encountered before. The main feature of the current situation is that there is an Internet network that can used via the Internet – services. One of the services most affected by the pandemic is education. According to the UNESCO monitoring, more than 100 countries have requested strict quarantine restrictions, which have affected more than half of students worldwide [1].

This work is devoted to an empirical study of the impact of the pandemic on students' daily life. The study was conducted during the graduation of students studying at the Faculty of Computer Science and Information Technology of Lviv Polytechnic National University for the specialty 122 "Computer Science",

© IFIP International Federation for Information Processing 2021
Published by Springer Nature Switzerland AG 2021
A. Byrski et al. (Eds.): ANTICOVID 2021, IFIP AICT 616, pp. 35–40, 2021.
https://doi.org/10.1007/978-3-030-86582-5_4

using Google Forms in 2021. The survey contained 10 questions on the impact of pandemic constraints on student learning. 159 respondents took part in the survey. These are students of the first, the second and the fourth years of study, including 93 first-year students. Most of them are young people aged 17–21. The ratio of girls to boys from 2 to 1. It should also be noted that the students of the faculty, in terms of selection of applicants, are the best graduates, the average entrance score for enrollment above 185 out of 200. Lviv Polytechnic National University started online learning on March 12, 2020. From that date, the Government of Ukraine [2] in response to the spread of infectious disease called for strict quarantine restrictions by preventing the spread of disease. The return to audit training took place only in a few weeks in September 2021. The purpose of this work is to draw attention to the significant transformation of the time spent on the computer of students during online learning, in relation to the sanitary norms established by the legislation of Ukraine [3].

2   Brief Publication Analysis

Despite the relatively short duration of the pandemic, there are enough publications to study the various effects of this complex phenomenon. Let us take a brief look at the ones we think are directly related to this study. In [4], using telephone interviews, a study of the impact of lockdown on the professional careers of university students in Bangladesh was conducted. Researchers noted a significant negative impact of pandemic restrictions on both the professional growth of students and the general morale. In [5], a survey of 59 respondents from Qassim University QU-KSA examined the relationship between student learning strategies and factors such as class schedule, access to classes, level of engagement in online learning. The study aims to find positive factors for the opportunity to offer better learning opportunities to students both during the Corona and in the post-Corona periods. In [6], the classification of the effects of various factors on the course of the pandemic. In [7,8], a survey of students assessed the perception of Polish students of the transfer to distance learning. The authors note the negative impact of the pandemic on the learning process and the well-being of students, especially freshmen. Paper [9] examines the impact of the pandemic on various spheres of life in 11 countries: United Kingdom, Belgium, Netherlands, Bulgaria, Czech Republic, Finland, India, Latvia, Poland, Romania, and Sweden. An interesting study of the perception of the pandemic by Polish society in 2020 based on the analysis of the content of posts on social networks is presented in [10]. The use of neural networks to predict the nature of the pandemic is presented in [11]. The [12] shows that the COVID-19 pandemic, and social stratification is growing: the poor are getting poorer and the rich are getting richer. In work [13], in order to improve the sustainable education basis on distance learning, a survey was conducted among both students and teachers. Paper [14] analyzes the advantages and disadvantages of online teaching, the level of satisfaction and acceptance based on a survey of high school lecturers. It has been shown that the pandemic has a significant impact on the digitalization of education. Paper [15] shows that the educational system in Ukraine is changing significantly due to the impact of the pandemic. The authors noted that along with the negative effect, a large proportion of changes are positive. Thus, it can be concluded that the scientific community of the world is actively engaged in studying the new phenomenon of the COVID-19 pandemic, which caused the crisis on the planet, and its effects on various parts of human life.

3 Student Survey Results

The questions for the survey were inspired by the fact that the authors, as high school teachers, felt a significant increase in the daily workload caused by the pandemic and the transition to an online form of teaching material. This has also led to a significant increase in the time spent working with the computer. This time significantly exceeded the norms established by law (max. 8 h a day [2] with a break of at least 10 min every hour). It was clear that the increase in workload for students is not less, but perhaps more. We would like to emphasize that the conducted research cannot be considered universal, i.e. one that reflects the situation in Ukraine in general, given that

(i) the number of respondents is insignificant (159 respondents in total);
(ii) students are a specific contingent in terms of age and preferences;
(iii) questions for the survey were formed by non-professional sociologists;
(iv) only 10 questions were asked. Nevertheless, we believe that the results objectively indicate the problem of the inability to control compliance with sanitary norms of computer time during distance learning.

Consider the answers to the question: "How much has the pandemic increased the number of hours spent at the computer per day?" and "How many hours per day has your time for self-study or study material increased?" The proposed answer options are a number from 1 to 10. The results are presented in Fig. 1, Fig. 2, respectively. We see (see Fig. 1) that 110 (69.1%) respondents believe that working hours have increased by 5 h or more. Moreover, 25 (15.7%) answered that this time increased by 10 h. Figure 2 also shows that if these hours are associated with learning, conciseness 88 (55.3%) respondents say that the time spent at the computer has increased by 5 or more hours.

Question "Has your budget spending changed due to the pandemic?" received the answer that the costs have not changed – 74 (46.5%); increased – 80 (53.3%); decreased – 6 (3.8%). Question "Did the pandemic affect your visits to streaming pages?" has answers that visits have not changed – 87 (54.7%); increased – 70 (44%); decreased – 2 (1.8%). 55 (34.6%) have feelings of insecurity in the future due to the pandemic. 135 (84.9%) consider themselves sufficiently informed about the methods of preventing the spread of coronavirus. The question "Has anyone in your family lost their job due to a pandemic" was answered "no" 122 times (76.7%), the answer "yes" 9 times (5.7%), partially 28 times (17.6%). Interestingly, the total number of unemployed (fully and partially) of 23.3% correlates well with the value of unemployment due to the pandemic of 22%, which was calculated by UNICEF experts in Ukraine. Among all 159 respondents, 73 (45.9%)

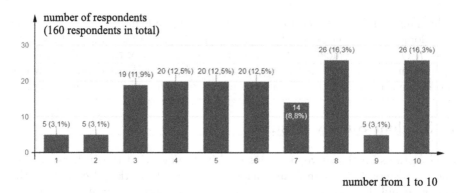

Fig. 1. Answers to the survey question: "How much has the pandemic increased the number of hours spent at the computer per day?" (160 respondents).

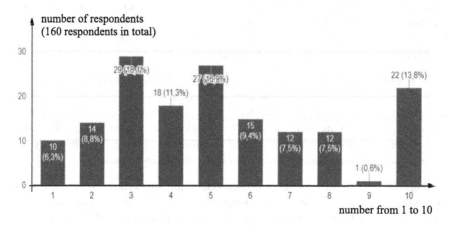

Fig. 2. Answers to the survey question: "How many hours per day has your time for self-study or study material increased?" (160 respondents)

believe that the number of online purchases has not changed, 80 (50.3%) has increased, and 6 (3.8%) have decreased.

The question "Which area of your life has been most affected by the pandemic?" received the following distribution of answers (presented in descending order): training – 114 (71.7%); rest – 26 (16.7%); work – 7 (4.4%); relations in the team – 3 (1.9%); for all of the above – 3 (1.9%); family relations – 2 (1.3%); the rest (relationship with the opposite sex, health) received 1 vote (0.6%).

When answering the last question: "What is most annoying about quarantine restrictions?" students had the opportunity to write their own answer. That is why we received such a list of things that cause irritation during the forced quarantine restriction of citizens' freedoms. The list is presented in descending order: lack of travel – 49 (30.8%); closed cafes, bars, restaurants – 35 (22%); wearing a mask – 29 (18.2%); closed cinemas 13 (8.2%); lack of concerts and music festivals 10 (6.3%); all listed – 9 (5.6%); indoor gyms – 4 (2.5%); closed museums – 2 (1.3%); distance learning – 2 (1.3%); destruction of sleep mode 1 (0.6%); disorganization of people 1 (0.6%); difficulty establishing a daily routine 1 (0.6%); quarantine restrictions 1 (0.6%); nothing annoying 1 (0.6%).

Thus, all 10 survey responses were analyzed and the empirical study was completed.

4   Conclusion

The study fully confirms the opinion of other researchers that the pandemic has a great impact on higher education. This effect is long-term and has not yet been studied. At present, the final consequences of the pandemic are absolutely impossible to predict. However, the study shows certain trends that show the short-term impact of quarantine restrictions, as well as the transition to distance learning. Adding to the optimism is the fact that the transition to distance learning has some positive consequences, which will probably be implemented in the educational process in the postpartum period. Among them is the constant access of students to methodical materials in the form of video lectures, presentations, or text methodical developments. Among the most negative consequences are the lack of social communication, an extremely significant increase in time spent working with a computer. An increase in the length of the working day and a change in the daily routine can be observed in both students and teachers. In the future, it would be interesting to conduct such a study in a next the 2022 year. It will be interesting to expand the list of questions in the survey, add more questions related to the professional orientation of students.

References

1. UNESCO: COVID-19 educational disruption and response UNESCO (2020a). https://en.unesco.org/news/covid-19-educational-disruption-and-response
2. The Cabinet Ministers of Ukraine Resolution on 11.03.2020 No 211 On prevention of the spread of coronavirus COVID-19 on the territory of Ukraine. https://www.kmu.gov.ua/npasearch?from=11.03.2020to=11.03.2020
3. Council, L.C.: Arrangement and equipment of computer rooms in educational institutions and the mode of work of students on personal computers (DSanPiN 5.5.6.009-98). https://city-adm.lviv.ua/news/science-and-health/medicine/219680-sanitarno-hihiienichni-vymohy-roboty-na-komp-iuteri-v-navchalnykh-zakladakh
4. Ela, M., et al.: Prolonged lockdown and academic uncertainties in Bangladesh: a qualitative investigation during the COVID-19 pandemic. Heliyon **7**(2), e06263 (2021). https://doi.org/http://dx.doi.org/10.1016/j.heliyon.2021.e06263
5. Odeh, B., Al-Sa'Egh, N., Qarabesh, M.: Corona pandemic and new educational interventions for Saudi learners: a socio-psychological study at Qassim university. Asian ESP J. **16**(52), 86–101 (2020)
6. Shakhovska, N., Izonin, I., Melnykova, N.: The hierarchical classifier for COVID-19 resistance evaluation. Data **6**(1), 1–17 (2021). https://doi.org/http://dx.doi.org/10.3390/data6010006

7. Cicha, K., Rizun, M., Rutecka, P., Strzelecki, A.: COVID-19 and higher education: first-year students' expectations toward distance learning. Sustainability **13**(4), 1–20 (2021). https://doi.org/http://dx.doi.org/10.3390/su13041889

8. Rizun, M., Strzelecki, A.: Students' acceptance of the COVID-19 impact on shifting higher education to distance learning in Poland. Int. J. Environ. Res. Public Health **17**(18), 1–19 (2020). https://doi.org/http://dx.doi.org/10.3390/ijerph171864

9. Georgieva, I., et al.: Perceived effectiveness, restrictiveness, and compliance with containment measures against the COVID-19 pandemic. An international comparative study in 11 countries. Int. J. Environ. Res. Public Health **18**(7), 3806 (2021). https://doi.org/http://dx.doi.org/10.3390/ijerph18073806

10. Domalewska, D.: An analysis of COVID-19 economic measures and attitudes: evidence from social media mining. J. Big Data **8**(1), 42 (2021). https://doi.org/http://dx.doi.org/10.1186/s40537-021-00431-z

11. Strontsitska, A., Pavliuk, O., Dunaev, R., Derkachuk, R.: Forecast of the number of new patients and those who died from COVID-19 in Bahrain. In: The 2020 International Conference on Decision Aid Sciences and Application, DASA, pp. 422–426 (2020). https://doi.org/http://dx.doi.org/10.1109/DASA51403.2020.9317122

12. Borodchuk, N., Cherenko, L.: Fight against COVID-19 in Ukraine: initial poverty impact assessments. https://fpsu.org.ua/materialy/18182-borotba-z-covid-19-v-ukrajini-yunisef-podali-pochatkovi-otsinki-vplivu-na-bidnist.html

13. Poplavska, O., Danylevych, N., Rudakova, S., Shchetinina, L.: Distance technologies in sustainable education: the case of Ukraine during the coronavirus pandemic. In: The E3S Web of Conferences, p. 255 (2021). https://doi.org/http://dx.doi.org/10.1088/1742-6596/1840/1/012050

14. Bakhmat, L., Babakina, O., Belmaz, Y.: Assessing online education during the COVID-19 pandemic: a survey of lecturers in Ukraine. J. Phys. Conf. Ser. **1840**(1) (2021). https://doi.org/http://dx.doi.org/10.1088/1742-6596/1840/1/012050

15. Lokshyna, P., Topuzov, P.: COVID-19 and education in Ukraine: responses from the authorities and opinions of educators. Pers. Educ. **39**(1), 207–230 (2021). https://doi.org/http://dx.doi.org/10.18820/2519593X/pie.v39.i1.13

How Newspapers Portrayed COVID-19
A Study Based on United Kingdom and Bangladesh

Redwan Ahmed Rizvee[1]([✉])(iD) and Moinul Zaber[1,2,3]

[1] Data and Design Lab (dndlab.org), Dhaka, Bangladesh
zaber@unu.edu
[2] University of Dhaka, Dhaka, Bangladesh
[3] UNU-EGOV, United Nations University, Guimarães, Portugal

Abstract. In this study, we wanted to see how as a representative of a society newspaper portrayed COVID-19. For this purpose, this study considered two countries United Kingdom (UK) and Bangladesh (BD), and analyzed how COVID-19 as an external event was focused in the newspapers. To conduct the analysis, we handpicked a set of covid related feature terms, and using Latent Dirichlet Allocation (LDA) we verified the coherency of the chosen terms. The main finding of this study is that, initially as a new event COVID-19 found huge importance in the newspapers, but with gradual time progression, this became a new normal event and lost its initial insurgence of focus and took a stable condition. We also observed that despite being quite different demographically, geographically, economically along with being affected differently due to covid, UK and BD exhibit quite similar characteristics in portraying covid in newspapers. The decisions were arrived at by applying different types of Natural Language Processing (NLP) tools and statistical analysis. For experimentation, we collected all the published news articles from two newspapers, the Guardian and the Daily Star from January 1, 2020, to March 31, 2021.

Keywords: COVID-19 · Newspapers' portrayal · Media response · Crisis communication · External event effect · UK · Bangladesh

1   Introduction

Due to severity and widespread WHO declared COVID-19 as a pandemic on March 2020[1] and the world is still not free from the grasp of the coronavirus.

This paper is a result of the project "SmartEGOV: Harnessing EGOV for Smart Governance (Foundations, methods, Tools)/NORTE-01-0145-FEDER-000037", supported by Norte Portugal Regional Operational Programme (NORTE 2020), under the PORTUGAL 2020 Partnership Agreement, through the European Regional Development Fund (EFDR).

[1] https://en.wikipedia.org/wiki/COVID-19_pandemic.

© IFIP International Federation for Information Processing 2021
Published by Springer Nature Switzerland AG 2021
A. Byrski et al. (Eds.): ANTICOVID 2021, IFIP AICT 616, pp. 41–52, 2021.
https://doi.org/10.1007/978-3-030-86582-5_5

SARS-CoV-2 is the virus that causes COVID-19 and responsible for the respiratory illness symptoms[2]. Since the appearance of covid, the world has been at a stalemate and almost each country has been facing challenges in different sectors, e.g., health, education, economy, etc. Each country's government has taken strategies to stand against covid based on their capability and covid situation's severity, e.g., lockdown, vaccination, increasing tests, etc. But how the society is reacting is another important challenge, e.g., support towards govt.'s strategies, awareness towards covid's severity, most dominating public concerns, etc. As a representative of society media can be very useful to answer these questions.

Newspaper has always been a very popular and affordable medium to express society's concerns, status, morals, policies, etc. and has been used as a good data source to conduct different types of opinion mining [9], to understand media response. Many literature have used newspapers to understand various effects of covid in society [9]. This study tried to find during this long period how COVID-19 was looked at in the newspaper. This study mainly focused on three important questions.

1. How society gave importance over covid.
2. Different types of portrayals of covid or which issues related to it were given more focus.
3. How covid's severity controlled media's. response.

Based on economical, infrastructural, demographical, geographical and other internal parameters each country can be broadly categorized into two groups, developed and underdeveloped. Our main goal was to observe how the answers to the above-mentioned questions vary for both types of countries.

As representative of developed and underdeveloped countries, we considered UK[3] and BD[4] respectively. From different aspects, e.g., economy, infrastructure, demography, etc. these two countries exhibit opposite characteristics. Also, COVID-19 affected these countries way differently. Up to now (May 30, 2021)[5], the total number of cases and deaths recorded in UK is around 4,480,945 and 127,775 whereas in Bangladesh is 797,386 and 12,549. In this study, we wanted to observe how UK and BD were affected due to covid and the associative response reflected in the newspaper along with a time series trend associativity between them. The main findings of this work based on the asked questions can be summarized as -

1. Covid as an external event was significantly highlighted initially. But with gradual time progression, the initial extreme highlight degraded and took almost a stable condition for both UK and BD.
2. Both for the developed (UK) and underdeveloped (BD) countries we found that similar issues related to covid were highly addressed.

---

[2] https://tinyurl.com/4dva2zaf.
[3] https://tinyurl.com/44yh63v3.
[4] https://data.worldbank.org/country/bangladesh.
[5] https://tinyurl.com/9st4ys9h.

3. The ratio of warning over comforting sentences was comparatively more pronounced and vivid in the charts for BD compared to UK in response to covid's insurgence.

In the following sections, we will discuss our data collection and analysis procedure and validate our findings.

2 Background Study

As a representative of society newspaper has been widely used as a data source for opinion mining to understand different aspects of society. In [5], the authors used topic modeling approach on the collected news articles to extract opinions of people about 'presidential election'. In [8], the authors used headlines to identify different types of sentiments through Support Vector Machine (SVM) based approaches. In [9], the authors showed how newspapers played a crucial role in development and adoption of different contract-tracing apps to fight against covid. In [10], the authors considered newspaper coverage to measure response to the covid19 crisis targeting New Zealand and Singapore. Their investigation showed that Singapore showed higher sentiment value compared to New Zealand in response to covid19 pandemic. They also showed the trends in mean media sentiment of different topics to understand their relative importance transition over their considered time period. So, newspapers have been used to analysis different aspects related to covid in literature. In this study, we wanted to observe the reflectance of covid in the newspapers within a time period from the context of developed (UK) and underdeveloped (BD) countries.

3 Data Description

As representative we considered two newspapers, the *Guardian*[6] and the *Daily Star*[7] for UK and BD respectively. Both of them are quite popular in their respective countries[8,9]. We collected all the news articles from January 1, 2020 to March 31, 2021. For each news article, we collected the headline, main news, URL, summary (if found), and publication date. For Guardian, we had around 14808 news articles comprising of 40625 unique words and for Daily Star, we had around 34995 news articles having 52775 unique words. The collected data can be found in this link[10].

4 Data Analysis

In this section, we will analyze our collected data from different perspectives and measures.

---

[6] https://www.theguardian.com/.
[7] https://www.thedailystar.net/.
[8] https://tinyurl.com/25ufnb8n.
[9] https://tinyurl.com/a87685ty.
[10] https://tinyurl.com/w7y6kdwv.

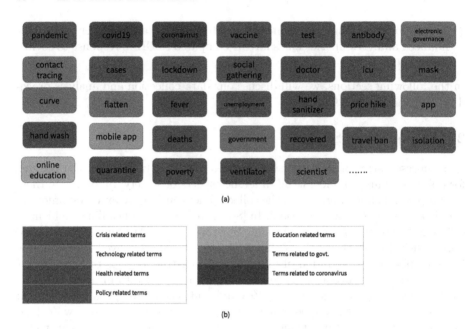

(a)

(b)

Fig. 1. (a) Some of the handpicked features with their corresponding category, (b) Color Coding to represent the categories

4.1   Validation of Covid Related Handpicked Features

We have constructed a set of popular covid related keywords (see footnote 10) for our analysis consisting of 175 core covid related terms based on different criteria, e.g., health, policy, crisis, etc. Complete list can be found here (see footnote 10). In Fig. 1, we have also shown a small subset of our handpicked covid related features as example. For each keyword we have shown a category which intuitively represents a reasoning behind selecting this feature as relevant.

To verify if the chosen keywords are properly selected to represent covid we have conducted an LDA-based topic modeling analysis [2]. For the empirically selected topic number, LDA provides a word probability distribution for each topic from the corpus. So, each sorted word probability distribution set represents the most relevant terms to that topic from the corpus. For implementation, we have used python's **gensim** library. The algorithm to find the topics using LDA can be summarized as,

1. First, we made a document for each news article merging its headline, summary and news. As pre-processing, we converted it to lower cases, tokenized, lemmatized and removed stop words from it.
2. Then we fed each document to LDA and based on the empirically set parameters it returned topics.

We have set $\alpha = 0.01$, $\eta = 0.01$, $pass = 4$ which are hyperparameters of the model and widely used. To find the suitable number of topics k, we conducted an exhaustive search by varying k between $[2, 10]$ (a popular segment) and finding the k with highest c_v score or coherence score[11]. We found $k = 10$ to give the highest c_v for both newspaper corpus (Guardian 0.55, Daily Star 0.52) and the topics were humanly differentiable. The top 30 words from the topic which represented covid in the Guardian and Daily Star are shown in Fig. 2 and 3 respectively. After finding the word distribution, we checked if our hand-selected core terms are properly representative of covid or not. We found that by looking at only the first 5000 words in the concerned extracted topic individually for both papers we could get 64% of our hand-selected terms in Guardian and 62% in Daily Star. So, the picked terms were quite relevant. Figure was generated using **pyLDAvis** library.

4.2 Guardian (UK) and Daily Star (BD) Discussed Almost Similar Types of Issues

To conduct this analysis for each newspaper, we merged all the articles into one large document. Then we removed the words which did not belong to our hand-picked features' list. So, finally We had a text document, which represented each features' appearance frequency in the collected news articles. Based on this, in Fig. 4, we have shown word cloud visualization for both newspapers. This visualization provides an interactive outlook to understand which terms have comparatively more occurrences. Using python's **WordCloud** library we exported the image. Seeing Fig. 4, we can get a grasp of the policies and center of focus for each country. From Fig. 4, we can see that both countries almost provided a similar type of focus on the concerned issues through more acknowledging them. Like here, we can see that both governments tried to impose **lockdown, travel ban**, focused on **social distancing, wearing masks**, etc. as prevention mechanism. Lots of talks about **cases, deaths, unemployment, doctors**, etc. as different types of crisis. Talks about different types of **apps**, collaborative **research** as technological aspects to fight covid, etc. In Fig. 5, we have shown charts for some of the found highly frequent words for figurative understanding.

4.3 Initial Highlight over Covid and Gradual Degrade in Focus

Now, we will try to observe if there exists any sort of relationship between covid incident occurrences (cases and deaths variation) and the percentage of appeared covid related terms. The main intention was to see if the variation of covid incident creates an effect on the number of appeared covid related terms. For this, we imposed two different y-axes, the number of covid incident data and the percentage of appeared covid related terms for each week (x-axis), and shown the results in Fig. 6. The main reasoning behind seven days as the unit is, if we look at patterns in the covid incidents, we will observe that the variation is not abrupt rather slowly upwards or downwards [3]. So, this window might help to better understand associativity. From the corresponding figure, we get

---

[11] https://tinyurl.com/9f36682d.

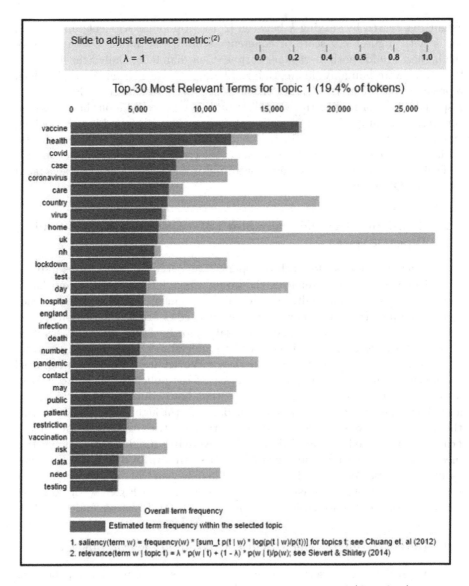

Fig. 2. First 30 words from the extracted topic as covid (Guardian)

similar types of findings for both of the countries. Initially, a significant uprising in the covid related terms can be observed. Mostly due to the new appearance of an external event, new sets of strategies development, news to educate people about this new virus, good variation in covid incidents, etc. But gradually this insurgence in covid terms gets reduced and takes a stable condition irrespective of good change in covid incidents. Mostly because it became a new normal

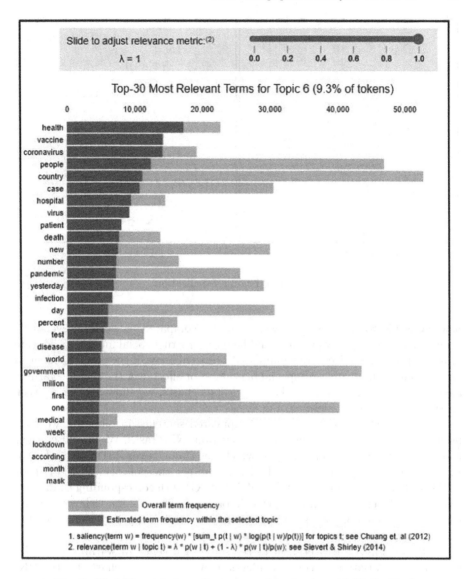

Fig. 3. First 30 words from the extracted topic as covid (Daily Star)

event and people already knew a lot about it. This summarizes the portrayal of newspapers towards an external event.

4.4 Propensity of Warning vs Comforting Sentences

Warning (or negative) lines mostly represent different types of concerns, negative vibes and emotions, fearful situations, cursed words, etc. and comforting (or positive) lines represent the opposite statements. The general characteristic of

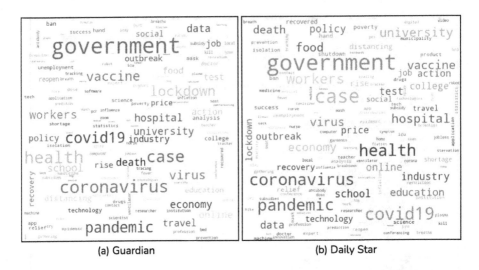

(a) Guardian   (b) Daily Star

Fig. 4. Word cloud visualization

newspapers is to show more negative events compared to positive events [7] because these attract people more and help to construct social morals, to educate or aware people, etc. Here, our main goal was to observe, if the covid incident as an external event creates any special biasedness or effect over the ratio of warning and comforting sentences. Similar to previous charts, we show a week-by-week analysis with covid incidents in Fig. 7.

To determine the polarity of each appeared sentence in our data we have used Flair [1], a popular framework to do various NLP tasks. We have used their trained model for sentiment analysis which was trained over IMDB dataset[12]. In Fig. 8, we have shown how using Flair, we can get the polarity (POSITIVE or COMFORTING and NEGATIVE or WARNING) with corresponding confidence score for each sentence and using that information from each article we identify the number of comforting and warning sentences and finally perform a week-by-week analysis.

It was our initial expectation to see some insurgence in warning lines (%) after upward variation in covid incidents. If we look at the charts for the UK, we can see some small variation (around 10th–15th, 50th–60th week) in warning lines (%) with the variation in recent (for that week) covid incidents but it is not too visible. But in the charts for BD, the visibility is quite vibrant and clear (around 10th–30th, 50th–60th week). A possible reasoning can be if we observe the incident charts of the UK, we can see that UK was comparatively more affected than Bangladesh with higher numbers. So, it is possible that throughout the year UK talked more about the negative aspects regarding covid, and thus when the insurgence in incidents occurred the ratio did not vary to a great extent.

---

12 https://ai.stanford.edu/~amaas/data/sentiment/.

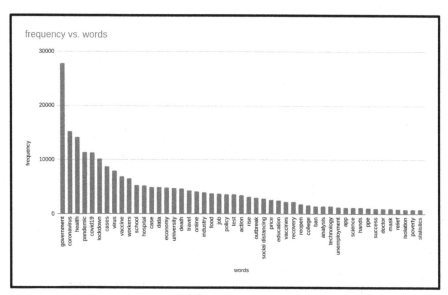

(a) Guardian

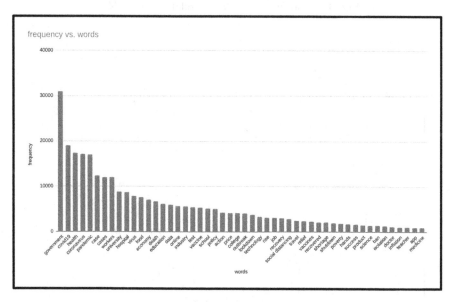

(b) Daily Star

Fig. 5. Frequency distribution of highly frequent top 50 feature terms

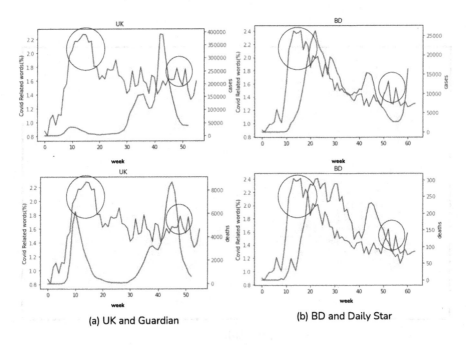

Fig. 6. Covid incident vs covid related terms (%)

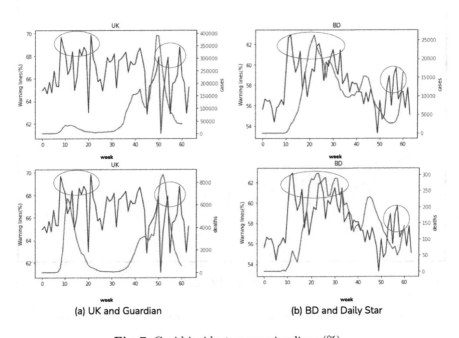

Fig. 7. Covid incident vs warning lines (%)

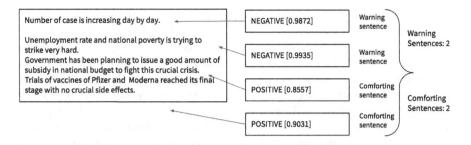

Fig. 8. Usage of flair to label sentiment of each sentence

On the contrary, it is possible that Bangladesh talked more about the negative aspects when the crisis was more dominant. So, the variation was more vibrant.

5 Summary

Based on the three questions which we have addressed in Sect. 1 and the discussion presented in Sect. 4 we can summarize our findings as,

1. **How society gave importance over covid:** Both UK and BD, showed significant importance initially which reduced over time with it being a new normal event.
2. **Different types of portrayals of covid or which issues related to it were given more focus:** Both UK and BD, almost similarly addressed the relevant issues.
3. **How covid's severity controlled media's response (Warning (%) vs Comforting (%) Sentences:** The ratio of warning over comforting sentences was comparatively more dominant with the variation of covid incidents in the chart for BD than UK.

6 Conclusion

In this study, we have shown how newspapers react to an external event initially and its gradual degrading trend in focus based on an analysis of UK and BD's covid situation and published news articles through applying different types of NLP tools and statistical measures. To summarize the intuition behind our findings, we can conclude as, the spread of covid and people's awareness or relative response did not go exactly side by side. People's actions are driven through different parameters and uncertainties. Covid created a significant amount of uncertainties and crisis in different aspects and layers of societies which have driven people to perform different activities where were not exactly helpful to prevent the spread of covid. So, the main point which can be taken by policymakers from this study is, the most important way to rise the awareness and support of people to fight covid is to reduce the uncertainties.

An important point to note is, the used mechanism to derive the findings is not exact. So, the findings can vary due to different types of data bias [4] and algorithm bias [6]. Also, to label the sentiments of sentences we have used a pre-trained model of Flair [1]. So, the biasedness occurred from the model is also included in the findings. In our work, we have hand-picked a set of feature terms that represented covid and used the pre-trained sentiment analysis model to conduct our experiments. As an ongoing work, we have plans to develop more compact strategies to discover a larger set of relevant terms and to design our sentiment labeling module to extract more in-depth knowledge related to covid from text data.

References

1. Akbik, A., Blythe, D., Vollgraf, R.: Contextual string embeddings for sequence labeling. In: Proceedings of the 27th International Conference on Computational Linguistics, pp. 1638–1649 (2018)
2. Blei, D.M., Ng, A.Y., Jordan, M.I.: Latent Dirichlet allocation. J. Mach. Learn. Res. **3**, 993–1022 (2003)
3. Dong, E.: Hongru du and lauren gardner. An Interactive Web-Based Dashboard to Track COVID-19 in Real Time, pp. 30120-1
4. Greenland, S., Mansournia, M.A., Altman, D.G.: Sparse data bias: a problem hiding in plain sight. BMJ **352** (2016)
5. Kang, B., Song, M., Jho, W.: A study on opinion mining of newspaper texts based on topic modeling. J. Korean Society Libr. Inf. Sci. **47**(4), 315–334 (2013)
6. Kuhlman, C., Jackson, L., Chunara, R.: No computation without representation: avoiding data and algorithm biases through diversity. arXiv preprint arXiv:2002.11836 (2020)
7. Luo, J., Meier, S., Oberholzer-Gee, F.: No news is good news: CSR strategy and newspaper coverage of negative firm events. Harvard Business School (2011)
8. Rameshbhai, C.J., Paulose, J.: Opinion mining on newspaper headlines using SVM and NLP. Int. J. Electr. Comput. Eng. (IJECE) **9**(3), 2152–2163 (2019)
9. Ta, T.H., Rahman, A.B.S., Sidorov, G., Gelbukh, A.: Mining hidden topics from newspaper quotations: the COVID-19 pandemic. In: Martínez-Villaseñor, L., Herrera-Alcántara, O., Ponce, H., Castro-Espinoza, F.A. (eds.) MICAI 2020. LNCS (LNAI), vol. 12469, pp. 51–64. Springer, Cham (2020). https://doi.org/10.1007/978-3-030-60887-3_5
10. Thirumaran, K., Mohammadi, Z., Pourabedin, Z., Azzali, S., Sim, K.: COVID-19 in Singapore and New Zealand: newspaper portrayal, crisis management. Tour. Manage. Pers. **38**, 100812 (2021)

Approximate Solutions of the RSIR Model of COVID-19 Pandemic

F. M. Pen'kov[1], V. L. Derbov[2], G. Chuluunbaatar[3,4],
A. A. Gusev[3,5(✉)], S. I. Vinitsky[3,4], M. Góźdź[6], and P. M. Krassovitskiy[7]

[1] Al-Farabi Kazakh National University, 050040 Almaty, Kazakhstan
[2] N.G. Chernyshevsky Saratov National Research State University,
410012 Saratov, Russia
[3] Joint Institute for Nuclear Research, Dubna, Russia
gooseff@jinr.ru
[4] Peoples' Friendship University of Russia (RUDN University), 6 Miklukho-Maklaya,
117198 Moscow, Russia
[5] Dubna State University, Dubna, Russia
[6] Institute of Computer Science, University of Maria Curie-Skłodowska,
Lublin, Poland
[7] Institute of Nuclear Physics, 050032 Almaty, Kazakhstan

Abstract. The Reduced SIR (RSIR) model of COVID-19 pandemic based on a two-parameter nonlinear first-order ordinary differential equation with retarded time argument is developed. An algorithm aimed to forecast the COVID-19 pandemic development by approximate solution of RSIR model is proposed. The input data for this algorithm are the cumulative numbers of infected people on three dates (e.g., today, a week ago, and two weeks ago).

Keywords: Reduced SIR model · Forecast the COVID-19 pandemic · First-order ordinary differential equation with retarded time argument

1 Introduction

In this paper we develop a reduced version of the SIR model [8] below referred to as RSIR model of COVID-19 pandemic announced in [6,10]. It is based on a two-parameter nonlinear first-order ordinary differential equation with retarded time argument. An algorithm aimed to forecast the development of COVID-19 pandemic by approximate finite-difference solution of RSIR model based on applying a perturbation scheme is presented. The input data for the algorithm are the cumulative numbers of infected people on three dates (e.g., today, a week ago, and two weeks ago).

The work was partially supported by the RUDN University Program 5-100, grant of Plenipotentiary of the Republic of Kazakhstan in JINR (2020), and the Russian Foundation for Basic Research and the Ministry of Education, Culture, Science and Sports of Mongolia (grant No. 20-51-44001) and the Bogoliubov-Infeld JINR program.

ⓒ IFIP International Federation for Information Processing 2021
Published by Springer Nature Switzerland AG 2021
A. Byrski et al. (Eds.): ANTICOVID 2021, IFIP AICT 616, pp. 53–64, 2021.
https://doi.org/10.1007/978-3-030-86582-5_6

The paper is organized as follows. In Sect. 2, the basic equations of RSIR model are given. In Sect. 3, an approximate solution of the model is constructed using a recursive algorithm implemented in Maple. In Sect. 4, examples of current situation are analyzed and some forecasts are discussed. In Conclusions, the results are summarized, the model drawbacks and prospects of improvement are discussed.

2 Basic Definitions

We recall the main definitions of our RSIR model [10] and relate them with definitions accepted in the conventional SIR model [8,9]:

$S(t)$, the set of susceptible individuals; $I(t)$, the set of the infectious (or currently positive) individuals, who have been infected and are capable of infecting susceptible individuals; $R(t)$, the set of the removed individuals not able to become infected (immune or dead); $N_{\max}$ is the population size; $s(t) = S(t)/N_{\max}$, $i(t) = I(t)/N_{\max}$, $r(t) = R(t)/N_{\max}$ are the densities, $s(t) + i(t) + r(t) = 1$; $\beta_L/N_{\max}$ is defined as the fractional decrease rate of the number of individuals in the susceptible compartment; γ_L is defined as the fractional removal rate of individuals from the infectious compartment; $\alpha_L = \beta_L/\gamma_L$ is the basic reproduction ratio.

With t expressed in the units of γ^{-1}, $t = \zeta/\gamma$, the SIR equations have the form [9]:

$$\frac{ds(\zeta)}{d\zeta} = -\alpha_L i(\zeta) s(\zeta), \quad \frac{di(\zeta)}{d\zeta} = i(\zeta)(\alpha_L s(\zeta) - 1), \quad \frac{dr(\zeta)}{d\zeta} = i(\zeta), \quad (1)$$

depending on *basic reproduction ratio* (BRR) $\alpha_L = \beta_L/\gamma_L$ as a parameter. Equations (1) should be solved with the initial conditions $s_0 = s(\zeta_0)$ $i_0 = i(\zeta_0)$ $r_0 = r(\zeta_0)$ and $s(\zeta_0) + i(\zeta_0) + r(\zeta_0) = 1$.

The main definitions of our RSIR model [10] are the following.

Let $N(t)$ be the number of infected individuals at the moment of time t, $\tau \approx 1/\gamma$ be the time, during which the infection can be spread by a single virus carrier. This time can be either the natural disease duration, or the time interval from the moment of contamination to the moment of the carrier isolation from the community. Here τ is a model parameter, $N_{\max} - N(t) = S(t)$ (or $(N_{\max} - N(t))/N_{\max} = s(t)$) is the non-infected population amount (or density) and $N(t - \tau) = R(t)$ is the number of people who have been infected previously, but are no longer infectious. Obviously, at $t - \tau < 0$ this quantity is zero, $N(t - \tau) = 0$. Then $N(t) - N(t - \tau) = I(t)$ (or $(N(t) - N(t - \tau))/N_{\max} = i(t)$) is the number (or density) of virus carriers at the moment of time t. Let $\alpha = \beta_L$ be the coefficient of contamination of a healthy individual as a result of a contact with a virus carrier per unit time (e.g., per day). This coefficient is defined as the probability of contamination in a single contact with a virus carrier multiplied by the number of contacts of a individual with all population members per unit time. In the present consideration, α is a model parameter. With the above definitions, $P = \alpha \Delta t (N(t) - N(t - \tau))/N_{\max}$ will be the probability of infecting

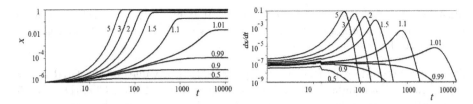

Fig. 1. a) Numerical solutions $x = x(t)$ of Eq. (4) and b) their derivatives dx/dt versus t measured in the units of $\tau/14$ at different values of $\alpha\tau$: 0.5, 0.9, 0.99, 1.01, 1.1, 1.5, 2, 3, 5.

one individual during a time interval Δt, e.g., during a day, for a given density of infection carriers. Then the number of diseased per unit time

$$\Delta N = P(N_{max} - N(t)) = \alpha(N_{max} - N(t))[(N(t) - N(t - \tau))/N_{max}]\Delta t,$$

gives a finite-difference equation for the time dependence of the number of infected and its continuous counterpart

$$\frac{\Delta N}{\Delta t} = \alpha(N_{max} - N(t))\frac{(N(t) - N(t - \tau))}{N_{max}}, \tag{2}$$

$$\frac{dN(t)}{dt} = \alpha(N_{max} - N(t))\frac{(N(t) - N(t - \tau))}{N_{max}}. \tag{3}$$

In terms of the density $N(t)/N_{max} = x(t)$, we rewrite (3) in the form

$$\frac{dx(t)}{dt} = \alpha(1 - x(t))(x(t) - x(t - \tau)), \tag{4}$$

independent of the total population and, hence, applicable to any community (country, city, etc.)

In Eq. (4), there are two model parameters, α and τ. Expressing the time t in the units of τ, $t = \zeta\tau \approx \zeta/\gamma$, we can rewrite Eq. (4) as

$$\frac{dx}{d\zeta} = \alpha\tau(1 - x(\zeta))(x(\zeta) - x(\zeta - 1)), \tag{5}$$

with a single parameter $\alpha\tau$, which within the above definitions represents the number of people newly infected by one earlier infected individual or *basic repro-duction ratio* $\alpha_\tau = \alpha\tau \approx \alpha_L$ Eq. (5) is shown to be equivalent to Eqs. (1) [5, 6, 10].

It is intuitively clear that if $\alpha\tau < 1$, then the number of infected individuals in the population will decrease, and if $\alpha\tau > 1$ it will increase, in full analogy with the kinetics of chain (nuclear) reaction. Note, that in Ref. [5] the so called logistic factor $(1 - x(\zeta))$ is set to be 1, which is true only when $x(\zeta) \ll 1$.

Equations (3)–(5) were analyzed in detail in our earlier paper [10]. The behav-ior of numerical solutions $x = x(t)$ of Eq. (5) and their derivatives dx/dt can dif-fer qualitatively depending on the basic reproduction ratio. For example, Fig. 1

illustrates this behavior at $\alpha_\tau = \alpha\tau = 0.5, 0.9, 0.99, 1.01, 1.1, 1.5, 2, 3, 5$, with t measured in the units of $\tau/14$. The derivatives dx/dt are seen to increase at $\alpha\tau > 1$ and decrease at $\alpha\tau < 1$.

Remark 1. According to Ref. [9], the possible known values of the BRR $\alpha_L = \beta_L/\gamma_L$ range from slightly above 1 for influenza, to 1.4–3.9 for COVID-19, 3–5 for SARS, 5–7 for polio, 10–12 for varicella, and 12–18 for measles. For COVID-19 these estimates of $\alpha_\tau(t) = \alpha(t)\tau \approx 1.4$–3.9 agree with the result of solving Eq. (3) with respect to $\alpha_\tau(t)$ [6, 10].

3   Investigation of the RSIR Model

Let us consider an approximation of Eq. (4) with the logistic factor $(1 - x(\zeta))$ set to be equal to 1:

$$\frac{dx(t)}{dt} = \alpha(x(t) - x(t - \tau)), \quad x(t) = N(t)/N_{\max}, \tag{6}$$

and its finite-difference counterpart

$$N(t + 1) - N(t) = \alpha(N(t) - N(t - \tau)), \tag{7}$$

where $\alpha > 0$, $\tau > 0$. The time variable t is continuous in Eq. (6) and integer in Eq. (7). Introducing a new time variable, $\zeta = t\tau$, we rewrite Eq. (6) in the form

$$\frac{dx(\zeta)}{d\zeta} = \alpha\tau(x(\zeta) - x(\zeta - 1)), \tag{8}$$

We look for the solution of Eq. (6) in the form

$$x(\zeta) = a \exp(b\zeta), \tag{9}$$

and arrive at the transcendental equation

$$b - \alpha\tau + \alpha\tau \exp(-b) = 0. \tag{10}$$

Equation (10) has two real roots, one of them is $b = 0$. At $\alpha\tau = 1$ this root is twofold, at $\alpha\tau < 1$ (>1) the second root is smaller (greater) than $\ln(\alpha\tau)$. To find complex roots, we substitute $b = x_b + \imath y_b$ into Eq. (10), where $x_b \in \mathcal{R}$, $y_b \in \mathcal{R}$. This yields the system of equations

$$x_b - \alpha\tau + \alpha\tau\cos(y_b)\exp(-x_b) = 0, \quad y_b - \alpha\tau\sin(y_b)\exp(-x_b) = 0 \quad \Rightarrow (11)$$
$$\cos(y_b) = \exp(x_b)\frac{\alpha\tau - x_b}{\alpha\tau}, \quad \frac{\sin(y_b)}{y_b} = \frac{\exp(x_b)}{\alpha\tau} \quad \Rightarrow \quad \tan(y_b) = \frac{y_b}{\alpha\tau - x_b}.$$

Let us look for the solutions with $y_b > 0$. For $x \geq \alpha\tau$, the left-hand side of the second Eq. (11) is less than 1, and the right-hand side exceeds 1. Then for $x < \alpha\tau$, the right-hand sides are greater than zero. This means that y_b should be sought

Table 1. Roots of Eqs. (10) and (13) at $\tau = 14$, $\alpha = 1/28$ ($\alpha\tau = 1/2$).

b	$\exp(b/\tau)$	z	$|z|$
0	1	1	1
-1.25643	0.91416	0.91875	0.91875
$-2.78900 \pm 7.43762i$	$0.70643 \pm 0.41511i$	$0.71978 \pm 0.40620i$	0.82649
$-3.35988 \pm 13.8656i$	$0.43135 \pm 0.65782i$	$0.45787 \pm 0.65116i$	0.79603
$-3.72088 \pm 20.2145i$	$0.09702 \pm 0.76044i$	$0.13483 \pm 0.76701i$	0.77877
$-3.98573 \pm 26.5360i$	$-0.23993 \pm 0.71295i$	$-0.19964 \pm 0.74148i$	0.76789
$-4.19505 \pm 32.8447i$	$-0.51868 \pm 0.52931i$	$-0.48985 \pm 0.58245i$	0.76105
$-4.36812 \pm 39.1461i$	$-0.68873 \pm 0.24785i$	$-0.68651 \pm 0.31959i$	0.75725
$-4.51566 \pm 45.4431i$	$-0.72036 \mp 0.07544i$	-0.75603	0.75603

Table 2. Roots of Eqs. (10) and (13) at $\tau = 14$, $\alpha = 1/7$ ($\alpha\tau = 2$)

b	$\exp(b/\tau)$	z	$|z|$
1.59362	1.12056	1.10950	1.10950
0	1	1	1
$-1.40710 \pm 7.42371i$	$0.78018 \pm 0.45740i$	$0.78945 \pm 0.44474i$	0.90610
$-1.97524 \pm 13.8578i$	$0.47660 \pm 0.72594i$	$0.50233 \pm 0.71379i$	0.87283
$-2.33548 \pm 20.2090i$	$0.10744 \pm 0.83950i$	$0.14806 \pm 0.84101i$	0.85395
$-2.60000 \pm 26.5318i$	$-0.26466 \pm 0.78720i$	$-0.21878 \pm 0.81311i$	0.84203
$-2.80914 \pm 32.8413i$	$-0.57251 \pm 0.58452i$	$-0.53708 \pm 0.63875i$	0.83454
$-2.98211 \pm 39.1433i$	$-0.76035 \pm 0.27380i$	$-0.75278 \mp 0.35048i$	0.83037
$-3.12959 \pm 45.4406i$	$-0.79534 \mp 0.08315i$	-0.82903	0.82903

for in the intervals $y_b \in [2\pi n, \pi/2 + 2\pi n]$, $n > 1$. When $y_b = \pi/2 + 2\pi n - \epsilon_1$, the second equation is satisfied by $x_b = -\ln(\pi/2 + 2\pi n) + \ln\alpha\tau - \epsilon_2$, where $\epsilon_i > 0$. We conclude that for $\alpha\tau < 9\pi/2$ the real parts of complex roots are negative, which corresponds to decreasing amplitudes of the oscillating solutions.

The solutions of the finite-difference Eq. (7) are sought in the form

$$N(t) = az^t. \tag{12}$$

Substituting Eq. (12) into Eq. (7), we get an algebraic equation

$$z^{\tau+1} - z^\tau(1 + \alpha) + \alpha = 0. \tag{13}$$

One of the roots is $z = 1$, at $\alpha = 1/\tau$ this root is twofold and the solution has the form $N(t) = a(t + c)$. Another positive root at $\alpha < 1/\tau$ ($> 1/\tau$) in smaller (greater) than 1. All other roots are calculated by means of built-in functions of the MAPLE system.

Generally, the roots of Eqs. (10) and (13) are related as

$$z \approx \exp(b/\tau) \tag{14}$$

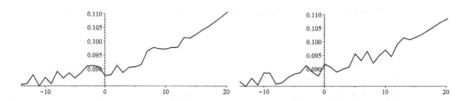

Fig. 2. Example solution of the problem (3) for $x(t)$ with oscillating behavior at $t \leq 0$

The calculated roots of Eqs. (10) and (13) at $\tau = 14$, $\alpha = 1/28$, and $\alpha = 1/7$ ($\alpha\tau = 1/2$ and $\alpha\tau = 2$) are presented in Tables 1 and 2. The positive roots z (1 and 0.91875 in Table 1, 1.10950 and 1 in Table 2) that correspond to non-oscillating solutions are seen to exceed all other roots by magnitude. Hence, the oscillating solutions decrease faster and can be disregarded (an example is given in Fig. 2). Note also that the equality (14) is satisfied with good accuracy, which allow using the finite-difference counterpart instead of the ODE.

Let the cumulative number of infected people $N(t)$ be known from official sources, e.g. [1,2], for three dates $t = t_0, t_0 - \bar{\tau}$, and $t_0 - 2\bar{\tau}$, where the chosen backward step $\bar{\tau}$ is an integer number of days. Based on the above considerations, we express $N(t)$ in the form

$$N(t) = c_0 + c_1 z^t, \tag{15}$$

which gives rise to a system of equations

$$N(0) = c_0 + c_1, N(-\bar{\tau}) = c_0 + c_1 z^{-\bar{\tau}}, N(-2\bar{\tau}) = c_0 + c_1 z^{-2\bar{\tau}} \tag{16}$$

with the solution

$$c_0 = \frac{N(0)N(-2\bar{\tau}) - N(-\bar{\tau})^2}{N(-2\bar{\tau}) - 2N(-\bar{\tau}) + N(0)}, \quad c_1 = \frac{(N(-\bar{\tau}) - N(0))^2}{N(-2\bar{\tau}) - 2N(-\bar{\tau}) + N(0)},$$

$$z = \left(\frac{N(-\bar{\tau}) - N(-2\bar{\tau})}{N(0) - N(-\bar{\tau})} \right)^{1/\bar{\tau}}, \quad \alpha = \frac{z^\tau(z-1)}{z^\tau - 1}. \tag{17}$$

Substituting (17) into $N(\bar{\tau}) = c_0 + c_1 z^{\bar{\tau}}$, we get

$$N(\bar{\tau}) = N(0) + \frac{(N(0) - N(-\bar{\tau}))^2}{N(-\bar{\tau}) - N(-2\bar{\tau})}. \tag{18}$$

Sequential application of this formula k times yields

$$N(k\bar{\tau}) = N(0) + \sum_{l=1}^{k} \frac{(N(0) - N(-\bar{\tau}))^{l+1}}{(N(-\bar{\tau}) - N(-2\bar{\tau}))^l}. \tag{19}$$

Expression (18) can be applied to predict the number of infected people $N(k\bar{\tau}) - N(0)$, while Eq. (19) should be modified for the finite-difference counterpart of Eq. (4), namely

$$N(t+1) - N(t) = \alpha(1 - N(t)/N_{\max})(N(t) - N(t-\tau)). \tag{20}$$

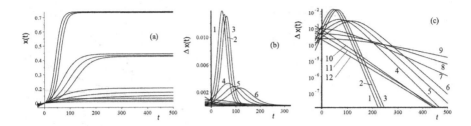

Fig. 3. Numerical solutions $x(t)$ of Eq. (4) determined by the current and two preceding values (a) and the corresponding differences $\Delta x(t) = x(t) - x(t-1)$ in linear (b) and logarithmic (c) scale. The parameters are $\tau = \bar{\tau} = 14$, $x(0) = 0.1$; the plots for $(x(-\bar{\tau}), x(-2\bar{\tau})) = (0.088,0.084)$, $(0.094,0.092)$, $(0.097,0.096)$, $(0.088,0.080)$, $(0.094,0.090)$, $(0.097,0.095)$, $(0.088,0.076)$, $(0.094,0.088)$, $(0.097,0.094)$, $(0.088,0.072)$, $(0.094,0.086)$, and $(0.097,0.093)$ are arranged from top to bottom in (a) and numbered from 1 to 12 in (b) and (c).

Using the perturbation theory, a slow variation of α can be shown not to affect the behavior of the solution $N(t)$ or $x(t)$ qualitatively.

Since α in Eq. (7) corresponds to $\alpha(1 - N(t)/N_{\max})$ in Eq. (20), in a rough approximation (18) yields

$$N(\bar{\tau}) = N(0) + \frac{(N(0) - N(-\bar{\tau}))^2}{(N(-\bar{\tau}) - N(-2\bar{\tau}))} \frac{(N_{\max} - N(\bar{\tau}))}{(N_{\max} - N(0))}. \qquad (21)$$

The solution of Eq. (21) has the form

$$N(\bar{\tau}) = N(0) + \frac{(N(0) - N(-\bar{\tau}))^2(N_{\max} - N(0))}{(N(0) - N(-\bar{\tau}))^2 + (N(-\bar{\tau}) - N(-2\bar{\tau}))(N_{\max} - N(0))}. \qquad (22)$$

Equations (22) and (18) provide upper estimates of the infected number $N(\bar{\tau})$. On the contrary, Eq. (19) takes into account the change in the infection rate by using $\alpha(1 - N(t)/N_{\max})$ instead of bare α and, therefore, can be used to determine the limit values. However, the resulting expressions are cumbersome. Therefore, the calculations should be performed for given τ, $\bar{\tau}$, $N_{\max}$, $N(0)$, $N(-\bar{\tau})$, $N(-2\bar{\tau})$. In this case, instead of calculating the limit values by Eq. (22), one can use the algorithm that follows from (20):

Algorithm:
Input: τ, $\bar{\tau}$, $N_{\max}$, $N(0)$, $N(-\bar{\tau})$, $N(-2\bar{\tau})$;
Output: $N(t)$, $\Delta N(t)$
1: Calculate c_0, c_1, z, α using Eqs. (17),
    and then $N(t) = c_0 + c_1 z^t$, $t = -\tau, ..., 0$;
2: For $t = 1, 2, ..., t_{\max}$ **do**
2.1: $\Delta N(t) = \alpha(1 - N(t)/N_{\max})(1 - N(0)/N_{\max})^{-1}(N(t) - N(t - \tau))$;
2.2: $N(t + 1) = N(t) + \Delta N(t)$;
    End of loop.

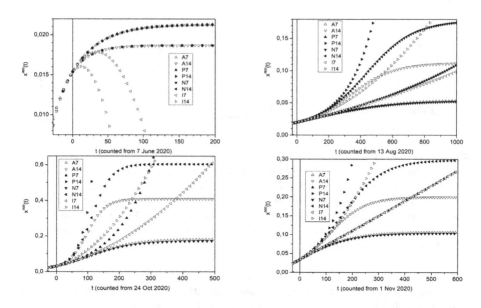

Fig. 4. Forecast of the number of cases (for $t < 0$, the values of $x(t)$ were calculated using the corresponding formulas) for Moscow, obtained using Algorithm (A), formulas (19) (P) and (22) (N), and interpolation formula (23) (I) for $\bar{\tau} = 7$ and $\bar{\tau} = 14$.

At step 2.1 it is taken into account that the value of α in (17) corresponds to the product $\alpha(1 - N(0)/N_{\max})$ in Eq. (20). Also, if $2N(-\bar{\tau}) = N(0) + N(-2\bar{\tau})$, then at step 1 we have $N(t) = N(0)(1 + t/(2\bar{\tau})) - N(-2\bar{\tau})t/(2\bar{\tau})$.

The described method allows the calculation of tables, using which from $x(0)$, $x(-\bar{\tau})$, $x(-2\bar{\tau})$ at $\tau = 14$ and $\bar{\tau} = 14$ it is possible to estimate the number of infected people $N_{\text{fin}} = \lim_{t\to\infty} N^{app}(t)$ and its maximum increment $\Delta N_{\text{fin}} = \max_{t>0}(N^{app}(t) - N^{app}(t-1))$ which can be chosen from Fig. 1.

The time dependence of the infected people density $x(t)$ at given values of $x(0) = 0.1$, $x(-\bar{\tau})$ and $x(-2\bar{\tau})$ are presented in Fig. 3. At fixed $x(0)$, the limit number of infected people is seen to depend on the ratio $\xi = (x(0) - x(-\bar{\tau}))/(x(0) - x(-2\bar{\tau}))$ for $\xi > 1/2$, i.e., for $\alpha\tau > 1$, when the daily increment initially increases. For $\xi \leq 1/2$, when the daily increment initially decreases, no such correlation was observed.

Remark 2. These solutions are fast-oscillating, with the period less than τ, and rapidly decreasing. For the finite-difference scheme the presented solution is general. If the main task were to solve the differential equation (3), then it would be necessary to make sure that there are no slowly oscillating solutions, even though it would manifest itself in the discrete model (3) as well. Hence it follows that when applying the scheme for a forecast, oscillations $N(t)$ should disappear. This will be illustrated by a comparison of the forecast given by the algorithm and obtained by replacing the quantity $N(t)$ with real data at step 1.

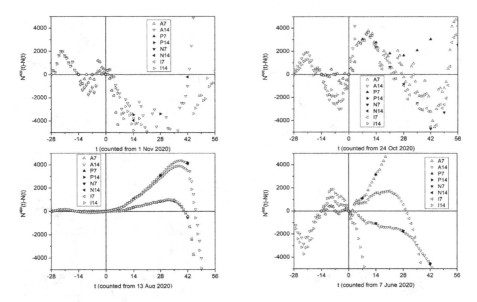

Fig. 5. Error in forecasting the number of cases (for $t < 0$, the difference $N^{\text{app}}(t) - N(t)$) for Moscow was calculated using the corresponding formulas), obtained using Algorithm (A), formulas (19) (P) and (22) (N), and interpolation formula (23) (I) for $\bar{\tau} = 7$ and $\bar{\tau} = 14$.

4   Examples of Current Situation Analysis

Thus, based on Eqs. (3), (16)–(17) and the assumption of the constancy of the coefficient of contamination α, an algorithm was developed and Eqs. (18)–(19) and (22) were obtained for forecasting. For a short-term forecast, one can use simple interpolation formulas

$$N(t) = N(0) + (3N(0) - 4N(-\bar{\tau}) + N(-2\bar{\tau}))(t/\bar{\tau})/2$$
$$+ (N(0) - 2N(-\bar{\tau}) + N(-2\bar{\tau}))(t/\bar{\tau})^2/2. \qquad (23)$$

Note that the parameter τ is involved only in the algorithm and does not enter the resulting expressions. Neglecting the change in $(1 - N(t)/N_{\max})$ at step **2.1** of the Algorithm, using (15), (17) we get $\Delta N(t) \sim \alpha(N(t) - N(t-\tau)) \sim z^t(z-1)$. Taking into account the factor $(1 - N(t)/N_{\max})$ gives a decrease in $N(t)$ for $t = 1, ..., \tau$, and then the product $\alpha(N(t) - N(t-\tau))$; the less τ, the stronger this decrease. Since $(1 - N(t)/N_{\max})$ changes by parts of a percent during the month, the discrepancies in calculations using the Algorithm for different τ will be small in the short-term forecast.

Figures 4, 5 and 6 illustrate the application of the proposed approach.

In Fig. 6, the data for Masovian Voivodeship (Poland), Moscow, New York and Peru are considered as an example. Beside the data availability, the choice of examples was motivated by the requirement that either the entire region

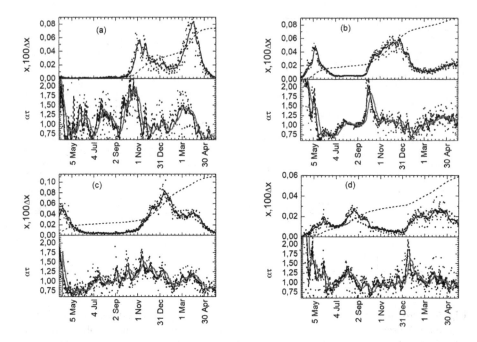

Fig. 6. Coronavirus data for Masovian Voivodeship, Poland (a), Moscow (b), New York (c) and Peru (d) during the time from April 6, 2020 to May 31, 2021. Top: number of cases $N(t)$ (dotted line), daily increase $\Delta N(t) = N(t) - N(t-1)$ (dots), daily increase averaged over seven days $\Delta_7 N(t) = (N(t) - N(t-7))/7$ (solid line). Bottom: parameter $\alpha\tau$ calculated from Eq. (3) (dots), its average over 7 days $(\sum_{i=-\bar{\tau}+1}^{0}(\alpha_\tau(t_0 + i)))/\bar{\tau}$, calculated from Eq. (20) with $\bar{\tau} = 7$ (solid black line) and $\bar{\tau} = 14$ (solid gray line).

(Moscow, New York) or it center (Masovian Voivodeship, Peru) should have a high population density.

Figure 4 presents examples of forecasting the number of cases $x(t) = N(t)/N_{\max}$, $t > t_0$ in Moscow using the data of Fig. 6b and four different values of initial time t_0 in increasing order. On June 7, $\Delta x(t)$ demonstrated a fall and α_τ has just passed the maximum point. On August 13 $\Delta x(t)$ was stable and α_τ has also just passed the maximum point. On October 24 the growth of $\Delta x(t)$ was observed and α_τ has just passed the minimum point. On November 1 $\Delta x(t)$ was growing and α_τ slightly increased compared to October 24. For the same backward step $\bar{\tau}$, the forecasts of the Algorithm and Eq. (22) commonly coincide with each other and with the forecast of Eq. (19) for $N(t)/N_{\max} \ll 1$, but differ from the forecasts obtained by interpolation (23). At the same time, there are no correlations between the forecasts obtained for different $\bar{\tau} = 7, 14$ and according to different interpolation.

Figure 5 illustrates the errors $N^{\mathrm{app}}(t) - N(t)$ in predicting the number of cases. The results are poor because in most cases the BRR $\alpha_\tau(t) = \alpha(t)\tau$ changes abruptly. Meanwhile, cases of almost constant little-changing $\alpha_\tau(t)$ have been observed, the longest one lasting half a month (August–early September) in Moscow. In this case, the forecast gave satisfactory results for about 40 days.

Of more importance is the evidence that the above algorithm and related formulas can predict disease peaks. As is seen in Fig. 6 for Masovian Voivodeship, Moscow, New York and Peru, the peak $\Delta x(t)$ is preceded by an increase in $\alpha_\tau(t) = \alpha(t)\tau$ above one. The value of $\alpha_\tau(t)$ was calculated from Eq. (3), its averaging $(\sum_{i=-\bar{\tau}+1}^{0}(\alpha_\tau(t_0 + i)))/\bar{\tau}$ for $\bar{\tau}$ days and from Eq. (20) for different backward steps $\bar{\tau}$. As $\bar{\tau}$ increases, the functions of the basic reproduction ratio $\alpha_\tau(t)$ become less oscillating, and for the same $\bar{\tau}$ they practically coincide, except for the peaks.

Remark 3. In solving the direct problem, the basic reproduction ratio $\alpha_\tau(t)$ $= \alpha(t)\tau$ is determined from a priori factors not considered in this model (humidity, temperature, social constraints, ...) and is time-dependent. An example of modeling dependence in the form of a smooth step function related to social constraints for March–April 2020 in Italy, describing well the current data, was given in Ref. [5]. In the approach presented here, we solve the inverse problem of calculating the function $\alpha_\tau(t)$ from the equation, using the known data $N(t)$ on the WHO website. Using the found functions we make a short-term forecast with the help of the proposed algorithm and formulas.

5 Conclusion

The proposed two-parameter model of the development of infection in the form of an ordinary nonlinear differential equation of the first order with retarded time argument is actually a reduced SIR model with a functional relationship between patients and carriers of the infection. This reduction maintains an optimal balance between the adequacy of describing a pandemic in the SIR model and the simplicity of practical estimates. The model allows solving both the direct problem (known the BRR as a function of time, find the time dependence of the infected density $x(t)$ with given initial conditions) and the inverse problem (for given $x(t)$ find the time dependence of the model parameters). This allows a quick forecast of the development of infection based on previous information on the statistics of the disease (see Fig. 6).

The results can be used for a short-term forecast, using the developed algorithm with Eqs. (19) and (22), which do not contain the parameters α and τ, and the interpolation formulas (23). They can be also used to predict the disease peaks. The corresponding examples are shown in Fig. 6. As is seen from Fig. 6, the peak is preceded by an increase in $\alpha\tau$ above one. The value of BRR $\alpha_\tau(t) = \alpha(t)\tau$ was calculated from Eq. (3) with subsequent averaging for $\bar{\tau}$ days and from Eq. (20) for different $\bar{\tau}$. Note that as $\bar{\tau}$ increases, the oscillations of $\alpha(t)\tau$ become weaker, and for the same $\bar{\tau}$ the results practically coincide, except for the peaks.

In the similar delay model of Ref. [5], it was emphasized that a reliable forecast has to take into account the fact that the official data of infectious cases are obtained by counting mostly the symptomatic cases, probably discarding other infectious cases which could transfer the virus even without symptoms or with mild ones. Moreover, the procedure itself, the realization times and the number of the diagnostic tests could affect the data of both the total number of infected persons and the number of recovered ones. However, since delay model relies on the infectiousness time, it does not require fitting of the data on recovered persons, which may be affected by systematic errors. The uncertainty of the data on closed cases would compromise the result for the SIR model. On the contrary, the theoretical prediction based on the delay model with a priori given time dependence of the basic reproduction ratio $\alpha_\tau(t)$ agrees fairly well with the data set for the total number of infected cases, as shown in [5]. It should be note that in contrast to the approach of Ref. [5] we did not use BRR with a priori time dependence in our algorithm.

Further development of the approach can include the methods of optimal control theory [7] with appropriate restriction conditions $N(t) \leq N_0 \ll N_{\max}$ to solve a self-consistent problem for both $N(t)$ and the basic reproduction ratio $\alpha_\tau^{\min} \leq \alpha_\tau(t) \leq \alpha_\tau^{\max}$. We also plan adapting some features of SHIR model [3] and SS'HIR model [4].

References

1. COVID-19 dashboard by the center for systems science and engineering (CSSE) at Johns Hopkins University (JHU). https://coronavirus.jhu.edu/map.html. Accessed 09 July 2021
2. Map of the spread of coronavirus in Russia and the world. https://yandex.ru/web-maps/covid19?ll=41.775580%2C54.894027&z=3. Accessed 09 July 2021
3. Barnes, T.: The SHIR model: realistic fits to COVID-19 case numbers. arXiv:2007.14804v1 [q-bio.PE]
4. Barzon, J., Manjunatha, K., Rugel, W., Orlandini, E., Baiesi, M.: Modelling the deceleration of COVID-19 spreading. J. Phys. A Math. Theor. **54**, 044002-1-12 (2021). https://doi.org/10.1088/1751-8121/abd59e
5. Dell'Anna, L.: Solvable delay model for epidemic spreading: the case of COVID-19 in Italy. Sci. Rep. **10**, 15763 (2020). https://doi.org/10.1038/s41598-020-72529-y
6. Derbov, V., Vinitsky, S., Gusev, A., Krassovitskiy, P., Pen'kov, F., Chuluunbaatar, G.: Mathematical model of COVID-19 pandemic based on a retarded differential equation. In: Proceedings of SPIE, vol. 11847, p. 1184709-1-15 (2021). https://doi.org/10.1117/12.2589136
7. Henrion, R.: La theorie de la variation seconde et ses applications en commande optimale. Memoires de la Classe des sciences. Collection in-8o 2e ser., t. 41. Palais des academies, Bruxelles (1975)
8. Kermack, W.O., McKendrick, A.G.: Contribution to the mathematical theory of epidemics. Proc. Roy. Soc. A **115**, 700–721 (1927). https://doi.org/10.1098/rspa.1927.0118
9. Lazzizzera, I.: An analytic approximate solution of the sir model. Appl. Math. **12**, 58–73 (2021). https://doi.org/10.4236/am.2021.121005
10. Vinitsky, S.I., Gusev, A.A., Derbov, V.L., Krassovitskiy, P.M., Pen'kov, F.M., Chuluunbaatar, G.: Reduced SIR model of COVID-19 pandemic. Comput. Math. Math. Phys. **61**(3), 376–387 (2021). https://doi.org/10.1134/S0965542521030155

Information Entropy Contribution to COVID-19 Waves Analysis

Iliyan Petrov[✉] [iD]

Institute of Information and Communication Technologies (IICT), Bulgarian
Academy of Sciences (BAS), akad. G. Bonchev str, bl. 2, 1113 Sofia, Bulgaria
iliyan.petrov@iict.bas.bg
https://www.iict.bas.bg/ipdss/i-petrov.html

Abstract. The beginning of COVID-19 pandemics was sudden and unexpected in terms of scale and symptoms, channels and territory of propagation in different countries. This article discusses the possible information theory contribution for analysing the waves of pandemics on the example of Bulgaria. Under conditions of uncertainty and non-sufficient statistics the simple and robust data-driven approach based on the concept of information entropy provides additional possibilities for analysing the dynamics of epidemic waves.

Keywords: COVID-19 · COVID-19 waves · SIR model · Information theory · Entropy

1 Introduction

System complexity and structural evolution are key issues for characterizing the specifics of dynamic systems in a large number of areas. The research of complex systems requires not only adequate methods and tools for treating and analysing the large volumes of data, but also a systematic approach for collecting and selecting of raw data. The sudden and unexpected outbreak of COVID-19 created unprecedented for many decades stress in all social sectors [8]. In this situation, it is a challenging task to develop models for long-term accurate prediction of pandemics evolution. The traditional forecasting approaches are usually based on deterministic extrapolation of general indicators and their average aggregated statistics often results in different prognostics about the dynamics of infections. Reliable statistics and consistent methods are critical for government policies and medical measures about "how" and "when" restrictions on mobility should be imposed, revised or lifted in all sectors, including education.

This research is supported by Bulgarian FNI fund though project "Modelling and Research of Intelligent Educational Systems and Sensor Networks (ISOSeM)", contract KP-06-H47/4 from 26.11.2020.

This study explores a research path based on information theory, entropy and agent-oriented analysis for complementing the general Susceptible-Infected-Removed (SIR) compartmental statistics [7] with additional macroscopic insight into the time-dependant and territory spread of pandemics [1].

2   Information Entropy

2.1   Competition Evolutionary Model for Shannon Entropy

The assessment of information entropy is performed by specific indicators with relatively simple mathematical algorithms at two consecutive levels. Traditionally, natural sciences (physics, computer science, telecommunications) use the information theory concept for entropy to assess diversity, uncertainty, and chaos [5]. In our studies we use the small letter "e" and capital letter "E" to denote "entropy" at micro- and macro-level. Also, to distinguish different indicators we use the first letter from the family name(s) of their author(s) in front of the symbol of entropy - for example, "SE" for "Shannon Entropy" [9], defined as:

- Level-1: transformation of the values of components' relative parts "p_n" (probabilities or weights) into results which can be defined as "micro-level entropy (individual entropy)" in the basic function "SE":

$$SE = -p_n.log_b p_n \tag{1}$$

- Level-2: summing of results of "micro-level Shannon entropy" "SE" for obtaining the cumulative indicator for nominal macro-entropy:

$$\Sigma SEnom = \Sigma_{w=1}^{n} SE(p_n) = -\Sigma_{w=1}^{n} p_w.log_b p_n \tag{2}$$

Shannon Entropy is usually defined in 3 basic formats: $log_2 p_n$ - with information measured in "bits"; $ln p_n$ - with information measured in "nats"; and $log_{10} p_n$ - with information measured in "hartleys". To frame the systems' evolution in the entropy concept we introduce a novel Competition Evolutionary Model (CEM). In CEM, the values of maximal cumulative entropy for configurations with equal (symmetrical) weights of components are defined as:

$$SEmax(sym) = \Sigma_{i=1}^{n} SE(1/n) = -n*1/n.log_2(1/n) = -log_b(1/n) = log_b n \tag{3}$$

To define the values of sub-symmetric configurations SE(subsym) are introduced the following parameters:

- number of Transition Interaction Steps "TIS", and size of "TIS" defined as $\Delta p(TIS) = 1/TIS$;
- Part lost by leader - "$\Delta p(LL)$";
- Structural Phases (SP) - configuration wit "n" system components;

In CED, the competitive interactions between the consecutively increasing number of "n" competitors form separate consecutive Structural Phase (SP) within which at each TIS the leader loses the constantly defined part "$\Delta p(LL)$" of his initial resource "$1/(n-1)$" which is redistributed evenly between the other equal competitors until the full equalization of all weights in the system "$(p_w = 1/n)$". To model a full evolutionary process, logically, we have to consider the following condition: $\Delta p(TIS) = 1/TIS \geq \Delta p(LL)$. For simplifying this presentation we consider $\Delta p(TIS) = 1/TIS = \Delta p(LL) = 1/100 = 1\%$. The starting values $p(start)$ of the leader and his "$n-1$" competitors are defined as:

$$p_{start(leader)} = \frac{1}{n-1} \tag{4}$$

$$p_{start(equalcomp)} = \frac{1 - \frac{1}{n-1}}{n-1} = \frac{n-2}{(n-1)^2} \tag{5}$$

In each SP_n the number "m_{SP_n}" of TIS is defined as:

$$m_{SP_n} = \frac{1}{n(n-1)\Delta p(TIS)} \tag{6}$$

The interim transition parts "$p_{transit}$" of the leader and hiss "$n-1$" competitors within each SP_n are defined as:

$$p_{transit(leader)} = \frac{1}{n-1} - m_{q(SP_n)}.\Delta p(LL) \tag{7}$$

$$p_{transit(equalcomp)} = \frac{1 - \left(\frac{1}{n-1} - m_{q(SP_n)}.\Delta p(LL)\right)}{n-1} \tag{8}$$

where "$q(SP_n)$" is the consecutive number of "m" in each SP_n.

Finally, all competitors are ending the serial of TIS in each SP_n with equal parts(weights) "$p_n = 1/n$". In this context, the symmetric and sub-symmetric macro-level configurations form a discrete path of the boundary of the maximum and sub-maximum levels of entropy in a scenario defined as "Equalization within each population" (Fig. 1). The system's balance can be defined as:

$$\left(\frac{1}{n-1} - m_{q(SP_n)}.\Delta p(LL)\right) + (n-1)\left[\frac{1 - \left(\frac{1}{n-1} - m_{q(SP_n)}\Delta p(LL)\right)}{n-1}\right] = 1 \tag{9}$$

The Maximal Shannon Entropy $\Sigma SEmax(sym)$ for each population is reached in the unique and fully symmetric configuration [6] when all components have equal parts or weights ($p_1 = p_2 = ...p_n = 1/n$) as defined in in Eq. (3) - $\Sigma SEmax(sym) = log_b n$.

2.2   Maximal and Normalized of Cumulative Entropy

Maximal Entropy. The Shannon Entropy is used in several areas (telecommunications, computer science, biology, economics, etc.) for assessing the diversity and uncertainty in different systems with a large number of components [3,4]. Therefore, the values of nominal cumulative Shannon Entropy $\Sigma SEnom$ for non-symmetrical configurations can be very different and have to be normalised if we need to compare them with other indicators - usually, the universal and dimensionless scale "0 to 1". Such normalization is achieved by comparing (dividing) the nominal cumulative entropy values $\Sigma SEnom$ to a selected level of maximal entropy $\Sigma SEmax(sym)$:

$$\Sigma SEnorm(sym) = \Sigma SEnom/\Sigma SEmax(sym) \qquad (10)$$

Multi-system Normalization. This approach consists to select some maximum level of entropy for a symmetrical system with higher number of equal components "n_{max}" and to apply it for normalizing all systems configurations (symmetric and non-symmetric) with a lower number of components "n" ($n_{max} > n$). It is useful for comparing systems with different number of components "n" - in the case of COVID-19, "n" could be the number of sub-national territorial units in different countries (states, departments, regions). The maximum level for such "multi-system normalization" has to be carefully selected - if it is to high the classification capacity of most of the normalized values will be substantially be reduced and the classification of capacity will be limited. This method is also useful for comparing different systems the dimensionless scale (0 to 1), but its major inconvenience is that so far in practice it is difficult to have a convention for such "n_{max}" and its universal level of "maximal entropy". In our opinion, a reasonable level for such normalization in the social sector could be a macro-state with 1024 equal components with results displayed in Table 1.

Table 1. Selected values of Shannon Entropy in the "log_2" format

n	1024	100	50	20	10	5	4	3	2	1
$p_w = 1/n$	0.0098	0.01	0.02	0.050	0.10	0.20	0.25	0.33	0.5	1
$se(log_2)$	0.01	0.0664	0.1128	0.216	0.332	0.464	0.5	0.528	0.5	–
$SEmax(nominal)$	10	6.64	5.64	4.32	3.32	2.32	2.00	1.58	1.00	–
$SEmax(normalized)$	1	0.664	0.564	0.432	0.332	0.232	0.200	0.158	0.100	–

Figure 1 includes graphical visualization of the continuous basic functions for individual entropies "se" in the three variants of logarithmic bases ($b = 2$, $b = 2.718$ and $b = 10$) and the respective functions of nominal cumulative, which after normalization produce identical numeric and graphical results. Logically, for all values of "b" the Shannon Entropy produces similar in shape and different in size structural spaces defined by convex parabolas.

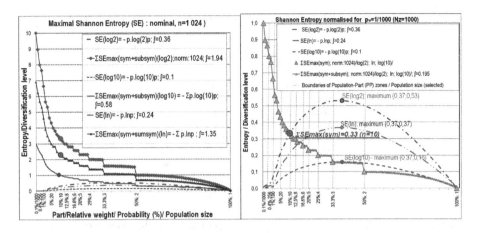

Fig. 1. Nominal and normalized cumulative Shannon Entropy

Single-System Normalization. To overcome some of the inconveniences of the "multi-system normalization" another popular method applies the opposite approach - the "single-level normalization" for each system with a certain number of components. Unfortunately, after such normalization all symmetric system configurations with equal relative weights ($p_w = 1/n$) but different number of components (n) produce identical maximal entropy $SEmax(sym) = 1$. By dividing the nominal (cumulative) entropy value for any asymmetrical system with unequal components weights ($p_w \neq 1/n$) to the maximal entropy value for this system we obtain the "normalized intra-system Shannon Entropy" $SEnorm$ as a convenient heterogeneity measure for systems with an equal number of components:

$$SEnorm = \frac{SEnom}{SEmax(sym)} = \frac{-\Sigma_{i=1}^{n} p_n . log_b p_n}{log_b n} \tag{11}$$

Although simple, such an approach is inconvenient for comparing systems with a different number of components but as it is frequently used in the majority of publications and for simplifying this presentation we apply it in this report.

3   Selecting Data for COVID-19 Entropy Dynamics

The purpose of this paper is to explore the most general issues of COVID-19 dynamics focusing on the basic trends and waves of pandemics development. Table 2 reviews the main statistical indicators available publicly in the official site of the Ministry of Health Care [2]. We observe all available information but as it is not equally consistent on national and regional levels we form a panel of 5 main statistical parameters - new positive tests/day, active (infected) cases, hospitalised patients, intensively treated patients, and lethal/fatal outcomes/day.

For example, except for hospitalized patients, a large number of "Recovered cases" are qualified as such on the basis of a formal expiration of the 10–14 day

Table 2. Selected values in Shannon Entropy the $SE(log_2)$ format

Parameter	Reliable	Transparent	Spread risk	National data	Regional data
New positive tests/day	Middle	High	Middle	Yes	Yes
Active (infected)	High	High	High	Yes	Yes
Hospitalized cases	High	High	Middle	Yes	No
Intensive care	High	High	Middle	Yes	No
Fatalities/day	High	Low	Low	Yes	No
Hospital free beds	Low	Low	Low	No	No
Recovered/day	Middle	Middle	Middle	Yes	No
Vaccinations	Middle	High	Middle	Yes	No
Infected medic. staff	High	High	Low	Yes	No
Age of infected	High	High	Middle	Yes	No

quarantine periods for "Active cases". Different test results seem not be equally reliable, but after confirmation they are automatically added to the "Active (infected) cases". Nevertheless, we retain them as a "first alert signal" and a useful wave indicator for COVID-19 spreading. "Fatalities" are the most sensitive issue, but their analysis would require detailed medical information and consideration of specific demographic factors in different countries, regions and social groups.

A major technical inconvenience for "New positive tests" and "Fatalities" is their volatility with chronic peaks on Mondays/Tuesdays and minimums on Saturdays and Sundays. As in many other countries, this is due to the fact that most clinical laboratories are operational only 5 or 6 days/week, and for that reason, these parameters are smoothed with a "7 day moving averages":

$$MovAv7 = (v_{t-3} + \ldots + v_t + \ldots + v_{t+3})/7 \qquad (12)$$

The 7 day period reflects reliably the infection period in which COVID-19 can be detected with high probability. On one hand, a 3–4 day period is not sufficient the smooth the formal distortions of data over the weekends. On the other hand, a 14 day observation period can reduce the possibility to monitor

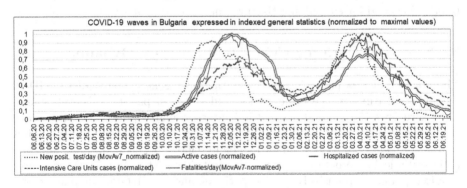

Fig. 2. COVID-19 general data panel statistics for Bulgaria (normalized to maximums)

the dynamics of spreading and implement adequate measures for preventing the effects of pandemics. This was the case in many small and big countries in the EU, but also in Brazil, India, Russia and the USA. The normalized to maximums results of panel indicators (new positive case/day - 3669/ 28 March 2021, active cases - 95442/ 7 Dec. 2020, hospitalizes case - 10649/5 April 2021, intensive care - 813/5 April 2021, fatalities - 140/27 Nov. 2020) are shown in Fig. 2

A very important issue in the COVID-19 crisis is the vaccination process, but unfortunately, its volume and speed in many EU countries are very limited due to organizational weaknesses in national health care services and delivery delays from vaccine suppliers in the whole period until May 2021. In this context, the reported problems with some of the vaccines led to unexpected demotivation and uncertainty among the population and health services. The information about the vaccination process was generalized mainly on a national level, and for that reason its entropy aspects could not be analysed adequately.

4   Nominal and Normalized COVID-19 Entropy

Under conditions of uncertainty and insufficient traditional statistics the entropy approach can provide additional possibilities for exploring the dynamics and spread of COVID-19. The signals from panel statistics can be supported with reliable information about the entropy level for the risky infection factor at sub-national, namely the "Active cases". Taking into account that in all countries the regional units have very different population in addition to the entropy assessment based on nominal raw data ("region by region") we introduce a second more objective indicator which is adjusted to the same size of population of 100,000 (100K) citizen, e.g. "Active cases per region of 100000 (100K) persons". The results in the formats of nominal cumulative entropy and single-system normalized entropy are displayed in Fig. 3.

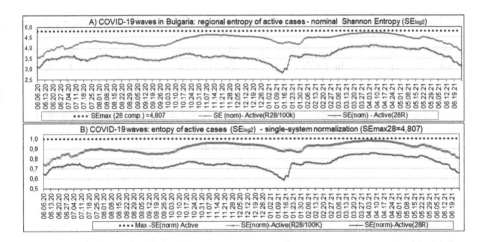

Fig. 3. Nominal and normalized regional entropy of COVID-19 spread in Bulgaria

The graphical analysis confirms, that the nominal and normalized formats produce similar profiles which values differ only in scale. In the two indicators, the profiles of entropies differ, since they are based on different sets of data. They provide a clear indication about three consecutive COVID-19 waves - two completed and one in the process of fading away in June 2021 when both indicators are slightly higher than the levels of June 2020. The first entropy indicator is based on official data about the 28 regions (*SEnom* and *SEnorm* "Actives per region") and produces lower levels of entropy, but at the same time with higher sensitivity and dynamics. This is easy to explain since the raw data set of relative weights reflects the information about the distribution of "Active cases" in different territorial structures. Actually, the largest region in Bulgaria is the capital Sofia with a population of 1.33 Million (19.2% of total population), and the smallest is Vidin - with 0.082 Million, (1.2%).

In the indicator "Active(28R/100K)" the population of all regions is virtually equalized for a basis of 100000 citizens (100K) to ensure a better comparability of results. Thus, we create a possibility for monitoring the spread of infection in a virtually homogenized environment. Such data driven abstraction allows to receive another objective view about the dynamics of pandemics and on an equal basis to explore in future other territorial (population density, social mobility) or agent-related (age, income, gender, health status, etc.) parameters.

Logically, after such equalizing the *SEnom* and *SEnorm* formats for "Active(28R/100)" produce a higher level of entropy with less volatility and these results are more reliable for considering the overall effects of pandemics. At the same time, the higher volatility in "Active(28R)" is reflecting the nominal intra-regional dynamics which is potentially very helpful as "alert signalling" for new waves that usually start from bigger and more active regions or cities and later spreads in the remaining regional units. As a result, the combined pair of entropy indicators provides a deeper insight into the available data and a double macroscopic vision for framing the duration of COVID-19 waves.

5   Increased Entropy in 2nd and 3rd COVID-19 Waves

At the beginning of the crisis, doctors and data scientists did not have enough experience to explore the COVID-19 data but later several approaches, methods, and models were developed and applied in different countries. One possible path of research is to combine the analysis of traditional time series that reflects only one parameter (mono-statistics) with time series for structural entropy which reflect the aggregated results for all the components (agents) in the system. In our case, the data set contains 28 data series for each of the 28 regions, which can be regarded as agents interacting with the infection. In this sense, the mono-parametric and entropy time series would be more useful if considered in parallel for analysing the evolution of pandemics waves.

In this report we focus on the territorial dimension of entropy and the spreading of infection among 28 Bulgarian regions. Figure 4 displays the attempt to capture and frame the COVID-19 waves with the aid of the two regionally aggregated regional entropy indicators for "Active cases" (discussed above, Fig. 3) and

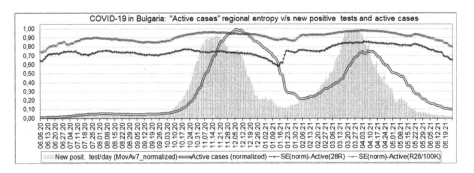

Fig. 4. COVID-19 waves in Bulgaria: entropy, new positive tests and active cases.

two of the five panel statistics - "Active cases" and "New positive tests" which can be associated with the genesis and the main processing risks of the infection in the SIR/SEIR models. Due to the very limited number of tests the 1st wave was not as dramatically reflected in the Bulgarian official statistics as in other countries. As logically expected, during the 2nd and the 3rd waves the registration of "New positive tests" precedes the accumulation of "Active cases".

The two entropy indicators reflect correctly from the start the specifics of all three cycles. In addition, the up-turns of territorial diversification preceded with 8–12 days the main traditional alarming signals for "New positive case". Unfortunately, in the spring and summer of 2020, this aspect did not receive due attention and analysis. Later, in each subsequent wave is observed a tendency for increasing of nominal and normalized entropy for "Active cases per region per 100K" above certain levels (in our case between 0.85 and 0.9). This is a reliable indication that the spread of infection is not linear or centralized and cannot be mitigated with liberal measures on a regional level. In this case, the entropy approach reflects the material information of virus spreading. Further, the rising of entropy levels above 0.90–0.95 reflects a diffusion type spreading and a danger of non-controllable chaos for a longer period. This is particularly true for the cases of intrusion of new virus variant that are characterized by accelerated spreading, longer recoveries, and more serious complications.

Regions and cities with open economies and active international and regional exchanges for tourism, work, business, and transport are particularly vulnerable to become the main gateways for more rapid spread of infections. In Bulgaria, this was the case for several regions and cities, whose population is more mobile in search of work or leisure recreations. In addition, the high entropy of "Active cases" can be regarded as an indirect indication about potential hidden channels of infections in areas with lower access and quality of health care services.

As a next step, Fig. 5 displays the attempt to frame the COVID-19 waves with two entropy indicators for "Active cases" aggregated on a national level and the other mono-statistical indicators from the panel statistics - "Hospitalized patients" and "Intensive care units cases", which can be linked with the results and back-end of SIR model. Here also, the first wave of hospitalization was not as

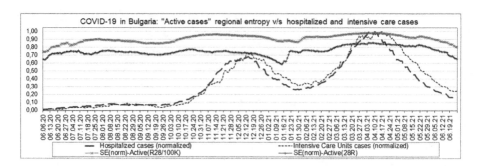

Fig. 5. COVID-19 waves in Bulgaria: entropy, hospitalized and intensive care cases.

clearly expressed as in other countries (Italy, Spain, UK). In the 3rd wave which started in February 2021 the "hospitalizations" and "fatalities" registered new record maximums in parallel with the highest entropy levels. These results can be interpreted as a confirmation, that the new mutations of the Coronavirus have more serious effects, taking into account that during the 2nd and the 3rd waves Bulgaria was dominated by the "British variant" of the virus. This observation is particularly valuable in the light of the possible rabid spreading of the Indian ("delta") variant of the virus in the summer of 2021.

The minimum and maximum values of the two entropy indicators and the five panel statistics allow to compare and analyse the duration periods of COVID-19 waves in Table 3:

Table 3. Selected values of Shannon Entropy in $SE(log_2)$ format

Wave	Indicators	Start	Min	Peak	Max	End	Min	Duration
1st	$SE(norm)/region$	6-6-20	0.644	7-8-20	0.759	25-9-20	0.706	99 days
	$SE(norm)/region100k$	6-6-20	0.745	28-7-20	0.857	15-9-20	0.848	91 days
	New positive tests/day	6-6-20	41	6-8-20	227	15-9-20	133	99 days
	Active cases	6-6-20	980	7-8-20	5205	15-9-20	4402	99 days
	Hospitalized patients	6-6-20	147	12-8-20	861	21-9-20	718	105 days
	Intensive care	6-6-20	12	24-8-20	74	24-9-20	28	109 days
	Fatalities/day	6-6-20	0	4-8-20	9	20-9-20	4	104 days
2nd	$SE(norm)/region$	25-9-20	0.706	23-10-20	0.773	14-1-21	0.584	110 days
	$SE(norm)/region100k$	15-9-20	0.848	13-11-20	0.962	29-1-21	0.867	134 days
	New tests/day	15-9-20	143	9-12-20	3980	19-1-21	416	124 days
	Active cases	18-9-20	4402	6-12-20	95442	4-2-21	20496	137 days
	Hospitalized patients	21-9-20	718	14-12-20	7244	27-1-21	2818	127 days
	Intensive care	24-9-20	28	13-12-20	595	29-1-21	257	124 days
	Fatalities/day	20-9-20	2	4-12-20	140	27-1-21	30	127 days
3rd	$SE(norm)/region$	14-1-21	0.584	4-4-21	0.857	30-6-21	0.655	165+
	$SE(norm)/region100k$	15-1-21	0.867	4-4-21	0.980	25-6-21	0.804	160+
	New tests/day	20-1-21	416	28-3-21	3680	25-6-21	361	155+
	Active cases	4-2-21	20496	2-4-21	70919	25-6-21	28490	150+
	Hospitalized patients	27-1-21	2818	5-4-21	10649	25-6-21	4201	160+
	Intensive care	29-1-21	257	29-3-21	773	25-6-21	460	160+
	Fatalities/day	27-1-21	30	2-4-21	126	25-6-21	4	160+

Both entropy indicators for regional entropy of "Active cases" registered increasing maximal values in the three consecutive waves. This is evident in the gradual entropy increase of "SE(norm)-Active/100k/region" in term of normalized entropy values: 1st wave - 0.857; 2nd wave - 0.962; 3-rd wave - 0.98. At the same time, the duration of periods with maximum levels of entropy in each consecutive wave is also increasing: 1st wave - 2 weeks with maximum of $\sim$0.85; 2nd wave - 2,5 months (mid. Oct. - end Dec.) at $\geq$0.94. During the current 3rd wave the maximum level of entropy of $\geq$0.97 was reached very quickly (within the 1st week of February, 2021) and since than the up-turn phase duration was approximately 5.5 months. The down-turn phase in the 3rd wave was longer than in some other countries due to the low speed of the vaccination process and the more liberal social containment measures.

The duration periods of COVID-19 waves framed by the two entropy and five panel statistic indicators were between 91 and 104 days in the 1st wave, and between 110 and 137 days in the 2-wave. According to information until 21 May, 2021 the 3rd wave is still continuing and will be much longer than previous waves. In the 2nd and 3rd waves, the starting moments in the two entropy indicators differed by 10 days and they preceded the panel indicators with 3–10 days in the 1st wave and with 13–20 day in the 2nd wave. In the 3rd wave the entropy indicators preceded the general panel indicators with 10–15 days. The main reason for this is the fact that entropy as a structural parameter is able to reflect in real-time the dynamics of distribution. Although it may seem that the 3rd wave is about to end, the serious risks persist. The prediction capacity of entropy can be very useful for defining more adequate prevention policies and national an regional levels. The major advantage of entropy is due to fact, that it captures immediately the dynamics of diversification of the virus propagation instead of relying on the cumulative values in the standard indicators. In other words, the increase of entropy is a clear signal that the channels of propagation are getting larger which will result in more active spread of pandemics. In addition, we cane note that the larger spread of the two indicators between the 2nd and the 3rd wave was and indication about the more active propagation of the virus through the channels of major cities and regions which contributed for the worse results in the 3rd wave.

Within the 1st wave the maximum of $SE(norm)/region100k$ was reached in 71 days with an increase of 0.112; during the 2nd wave - in 88 days with an increase of 0,114; and during the 3rd wave in 62 days for an increase of 0.113. The increased entropy in the 2nd and 3rd waves can be explained by several factors: the winter period, penetration of new and more infectious variants of the virus, more liberal policies for social mobility. The record high levels of normalized entropy closer to the absolute maximum of "1" in Bulgaria during the 3rd wave can be explained by the domination of the "British variant" and the very liberal containment measures compared to other countries in the EU. The national responses to such challenging "natural evolution processes" as COVID-19 will depend for long periods on the specifics of socio-economic and psycho-cultural specifics in different countries, regions, and social groups. These specifics should be more seriously considered in the ways of reporting official statistics, defining containment measures and implementing vaccination plans.

6   Conclusions and Further Research

The logical combination of reliable research methods is a promising path for exploring more efficiently the dynamics and evolution of complex systems and processes such as COVID-19 and other pandemics. Under conditions of uncertainty, the entropy approach allows to add new dimensions in the exploration of insufficient public data and to obtain valuable macroscopic insight on the spread of infections on national and regional levels. Being based even on limited empirical data this study confirms that the data-driven entropy approach provides very useful holistic view and prediction capability for enhancing the analysis of COVID-19. Our findings confirm that at the end of the 3rd wave the infection is in temporary retreat in Bulgaria as in many other countries and continues to be a serious risk for public health, economic development, social stability, and national security. The robust entropy concept can be a valuable contribution for analysing complex epidemic processes and optimizing the activities in many areas, and especially in health care services, education, communications, energy, etc.

The improvement of publicly available statistics should contribute to developing more reliable models and justified policies. Future research can be enlarged on internal and international levels and will definitely include the analysis of vaccination results for improving the quality of comparative studies and the knowledge about COVID-19 and eventual similar and subsequent epidemics.

References

1. Bandt, C.: Entropy ratio and entropy concentration coefficient, with application to the COVID-19 pandemic. Entropy **22**(11) (2020). PMID: 33287080. PMCID: PMC7712116. https://doi.org/10.3390/e22111315
2. Bulgarian Ministry of Health: Official web site for Covid-19. https://coronavirus.bg. Accessed 25 June 2021
3. Golan, A., Judge, G., Miller, D.: Maximum Entropy Econometrics: Robust Estimation with Limited Data. Wiley, New York (1996)
4. Harte, J., Newman, E.: Maximum information entropy: a foundation for ecological theory. Trends Ecol. Evol. **29**(7), 384–389 (2014)
5. Jaynes, E.: Information theory and statistical mechanics. Phys. Rev. **106**, 620–630 (1957)
6. Jaynes, E.: On the rationale of maximum-entropy methods. Proc. IEEE **70**, 939–952 (1982)
7. Kenah, E., Robins, J.: Network-based analysis of stochastic sir epidemic models with random and proportionate mixing. J. Theor. Biol. **249**(4), 706–722 (2007). https://doi.org/10.1016/j.jtbi.2007.09.011
8. Li, Q., et al.: Early transmission dynamics in Wuhan, China, of novel coronavirus-infected pneumonia. N. Engl. J. Med. **382**(13), 1199–1207 (2020). https://doi.org/10.1056/NEJMoa2001316
9. Shannon, C.: A mathematical theory of communication. Bell Syst. Tech. J. **27**(3), 379–423 (1948)

Computing the Death Rate of COVID-19

Naveen Pai$^{(\boxtimes)}$ (iD), Sean Zhang (iD), and Mor Harchol-Balter (iD)

Carnegie Mellon University, Pittsburgh, USA
{nvpai,xiaoronz,harchol}@andrew.cmu.edu

Abstract. The Infection Fatality Rate (IFR) of COVID-19 is difficult to estimate because the number of infections is unknown and there is a lag between each infection and the potentially subsequent death. We introduce a new approach for estimating the IFR by first estimating the entire sequence of daily infections. Unlike prior approaches, we incorporate existing data on the number of daily COVID-19 tests into our estimation; knowing the test rates helps us estimate the ratio between the number of cases and the number of infections. Also unlike prior approaches, rather than determining a constant lag from studying a group of patients, we treat the lag as a random variable, whose parameters we determine empirically by fitting our infections sequence to the sequence of deaths. Our approach allows us to narrow our estimation to smaller time intervals in order to observe how the IFR changes over time. We analyze a 250 day period starting on March 1, 2020. We estimate that the IFR in the U.S. decreases from a high of 0.68% down to 0.24% over the course of this time period. We also provide IFR and lag estimates for Italy, Denmark, and the Netherlands, all of which also exhibit decreasing IFRs but to different degrees.

1 Introduction

The COVID-19 pandemic has raged for over a year now, greatly disrupting the lives of people all over the world. While much research has been done on modeling the spread of the disease, one particular question that remains unresolved is: *What is the death rate of COVID-19?*

A good estimate for the death rate could better inform government policies, but it has been surprisingly difficult to estimate the death rate [5]. When we talk about the "death rate" we will be talking about the probability that an infected person ends up dying. This is formally called the Infection Fatality Rate (IFR) and will be defined in Sect. 3.

This research was supported by NSF-CMMI-1938909, NSF-CSR-1763701, and a Google 2020 Faculty Research Award.

A. Byrski et al. (Eds.): ANTICOVID 2021, IFIP AICT 616, pp. 77–94, 2021.
https://doi.org/10.1007/978-3-030-86582-5_8

1.1   Challenges in Estimating the Death Rate

Several challenges arise in estimating the death rate. These include:

Cases Are Recorded, Not Infections: Estimating the death rate requires knowing the number of deaths relative to the number of infections. Unfortunately, what is reported is the number of daily cases, not the number of daily infections. Note that a *case* is a test that results in a positive, however not all infected people are necessarily tested. Thus, determining the death rate firstly involves creating some *estimate* of the number of infections. One might think that testing can provide such an estimate, but testing is not randomized [19], so the proportion of test-takers who are infected is not indicative of the infection rate in the overall population.

Lag Between Cases and Deaths: In this paper we refer to the time between when a person tests positive (a *case*) and the potentially subsequent death as the *lag time*[1]. Unfortunately, this lag time varies for each individual. To make matters worse, lag time is also affected by larger trends, such as the age group that is most commonly infected and the treatments that are available [9]. Thus, the mean lag time may change as the pandemic progresses.

The Testing Rate is Not Constant: The number of daily cases can provide insight into the number of infections. However, the number of cases also depends on the rate at which people get tested for COVID. Higher testing rates lead to more cases being observed. The fact that the testing rate has varied greatly over time [14] makes it difficult to interpret the number of cases.

The Death Rate Varies over Time: The death rate is itself not constant over time. The death rate goes down when hospitals find new treatments, but then it shoots back up when hospitals get overloaded and run out of workers, oxygen, or ventilators [4]. The death rate grows when older people in nursing homes are being most commonly infected, but shrinks when younger people are most commonly infected [4]. Because the death rate varies, simply trying to fit one number to all the data is not necessarily the best approach.

Reported Numbers Are Not Always Accurate: Finally, we are always dealing with reported numbers, not true numbers. It is well known that in many states there is a delay in recording deaths and reporting them [10]. Some COVID cases never get reported at all. For example, a person may die from COVID without ever being tested [20]. Finally, there are both false positives and false negatives in the reported cases [8].

Antibodies Can Wear Off: People who were infected and recovered may lose their antibodies after a few months [1]. This makes it difficult to use antibody studies to estimate how many people have been infected by COVID.

---

[1] In some literature, *lag* is described as the time from initial infection to death, but such studies involve only a small group of patients, for whom the initial infection time is approximately known. In general it is impossible to ascertain the time of the initial infection from large-scale reports.

1.2   Prior Approaches to Estimating the Death Rate

There has been some prior work on determining the death rate, either within the U.S., or in other countries (see Sect. 2 for details). Much of the prior work is not actually looking at the Infection Fatality Rate (IFR), but rather at the Case Fatality Rate (CFR), which is the fraction of positive cases that result in deaths. Our goal in this paper is to determine the IFR.

For those works that do directly try to measure the IFR, most follow this simplistic 2-step approach which is not time-dependent:

1. Estimate the total number of infections by time t by looking at the results of antibody tests at time t.
2. Divide the total number of deaths by time t (this is easily found in reports) by the total number of infections by time t from the previous step. This yields the estimated death rate during the period $[0, t]$.

Sometimes the authors go a step further, by incorporating a lag between the case and death (or the infection and death). But this lag is often assumed to be a *fixed* constant value, estimated via small *in-person* studies.

1.3   Drawbacks of the Prior Approaches

There are several drawbacks to prior approaches. Firstly, the prior approaches are people-intensive, which is costly. Secondly, the prior approaches are limited in what they can produce. The IFR can only be estimated on days when an antibody study was conducted. To make matters worse, antibody studies become less accurate over time, since people lose antibodies, causing an underestimate of past infections [1]. But the biggest drawback of the prior work is that it doesn't take into account the changes in the pandemic. As we've explained, the lag time changes over time. The IFR itself changes over time. Prior approaches are not well-suited to take these temporal changes into account.

1.4   A New Data-Driven Approach to Estimating the Death Rate

In this paper we present a data-driven approach. Unlike prior approaches, our method does not rely on having a set of patients whom we can track and study. Instead, our approach is solely based on studying readily available numbers on *Our World in Data* [7] along with a single antibody study that can be conducted at an arbitrary time. By relying on a single antibody study, we can ignore later antibody studies which underestimate infections due to antibodies fading. Secondly, our approach easily admits temporal changes; in particular, we incorporate changes in the lag distribution, changes in the testing rate, and a time-varying IFR. The data that we use includes the sequence of daily deaths, daily cases, and daily tests, over a period of 250 days beginning with March 1, 2020, as well as antibody results that were available two or three months after March 1, 2020.

Our first key idea is that we need to estimate the entire sequence of daily infections. The sequence itself is needed because it allows us to see how the IFR changes over time and to study the temporal changes in the lag time distribution.

Our second key idea is that the sequence of daily infections can be approximated using a function of both the daily cases and tests. This function is increasing with respect to the number of cases but decreasing with respect to the number of tests. It furthermore assumes that a person who is infected is more likely to get tested than a person who is not infected. Section 4 explains the intuition behind our function. We find that the appropriate parameters of the function can be determined empirically via antibody results.

Once we have our estimated infection sequence, our next key idea is that we should determine the lag time *and* the IFR *concurrently*, not individually. Every possible choice of lag time can be viewed as a time shift of the infection sequence, while every possible choice of the IFR can be viewed as a vertical scaling of the infection sequence. Together, every choice of lag time and IFR results in a particular "candidate" death sequence. To find the "best" choice of lag time and IFR, we simply pick the parameters which result in a candidate death sequence which best fits the given death sequence in our data. We actually take this idea a step further and allow the lag time to follow a *distribution* whose parameters are incorporated in the above optimization process.

Our final idea is that this entire optimization process is best done by segmenting time into intervals (we use intervals of 50 days), because we find that the IFR and the lag time change over time. We repeat the above approach over several different countries, starting with the U.S. and moving on to Italy, Denmark, and the Netherlands. There is no reason why our approach can't be applied to other countries as well, provided that the data is available.

1.5   Synopsis of Our Findings

Figure 1 illustrates a synopsis of our findings for the United States. In Fig. 1(a), we see the sequence of daily cases (in blue), and above it we see our estimated daily infection sequence (in purple). Importantly, our estimated daily infection sequence is *not* a mere vertical scaling. The reason why is that in deriving our infection sequence we incorporate the time-varying testing rate, not shown here (see Sect. 7).

In Fig. 1(b), we illustrate our best "candidate" death sequence (which we derive from our estimated infection sequence as described in Sect. 4), and we compare it with the true death sequence. These two sequences are a good fit, indicating that our estimated IFR and lag are accurate. We annotate the top of Fig. 1(b) with our estimated IFR and the lag distribution in days for each 50-day interval. We find that the IFR decreases over time, eventually changing from 0.68% to 0.24%. We find that the lag is well fit by a Uniform(a, b) distribution, with a mean lag of about 8 days throughout the pandemic. Section 7 contains more details and also repeats this process for Italy, Denmark, and the Netherlands.

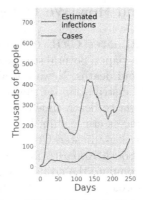

(a) Cases (blue) and Estimated infections (purple)

IFR	0.68%	0.60%	0.24%	0.30%	0.24%
Lag ~ Unif(a,b)	(2,13)	(3,12)	(7,11)	(7,11)	(8,11)

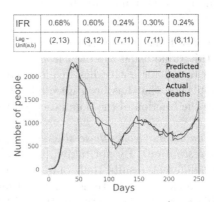

(b) Predicted Deaths (purple) and Actual Deaths (black)

Fig. 1. From cases to estimated infections to predicted IFR and lag in the U.S. (Color figure online)

1.6   Road Map for the Rest of the Paper

Section 2 discusses the prior work in more detail. In Sect. 3 we provide definitions and notation. Section 4 describes how we estimate a sequence of daily infections based on reported sequences for daily cases, tests, and deaths. In Sect. 5 we present our algorithm for calculating the IFR and lag time, and in Sect. 6 we refine our algorithm to look at smaller time intervals. In Sect. 7, we apply our approach to various countries. We conclude in Sect. 8 and discuss opportunities for future work.

2   Prior Work and How We Differ

Most prior work estimates CFR, the case fatality rate, rather than IFR, which is the focus of this paper. Several studies estimate the CFR while adjusting for lag between cases and deaths. Newall et al. [18] estimates the lag-adjusted CFR using a lognormal distribution for the lag with mean 14.5 days, which was estimated using the onset to death time of 34 patients, based on the case data from the Diamond Princess cruise ship. Using a very similar approach, Russell et al. [21] estimates the lag-adjusted CFR in South Korea. They used the first 66 deaths reported in South Korea to fit a lognormal distribution for the lag, which is then used to compute the adjusted CFR.

By contrast our approach does not need the data of individual patients: we estimate the lag distribution using the sequence of cases and deaths only, which allows us to make use of a larger amount of data from different regions. We find that assuming lag to be uniformly distributed yields a slightly better fit in our model than assuming a lognormal distribution.

Prior Work on Estimating IFR: Regarding IFR, various studies attempt to estimate this value using the data from antibody studies, in which a group of patients is tested for antibodies in an attempt to estimate the fraction of the total population that has been infected. The IFR is then estimated as the ratio between the fraction of the population that died and the fraction that was infected.

However, *unlike our work, these studies do not incorporate knowledge of the time-varying testing rate.* By not taking into account the testing rate, they end up with very different results than ours. Meyerowitz-Katz et al. [17] gives a comprehensive review of such studies which estimate the IFR. In particular, one study by Villa et al. [22] estimates an IFR of 1.1% for Italy up to the end of March 2020. By contrast, our estimated IFR for Italy is 2.2% around March 2020.

Several studies, e.g., Levin et al. [15] and Marra and Quartin [16], take lag into account in determining the IFR, but they assume a *fixed lag*. By contrast, our work assumes a *lag distribution* with parameters that can vary by region and by time. Our more flexible approach accounts for differences in the spread and reporting of the disease.

3   Definitions and Notation

Throughout this document, the terms *death rate* and *infection fatality rate (IFR)* are synonymous and are defined as follows: Consider a period of time $t \in [a, b]$, where a and b denote particular days. We consider the infections that occur during $[a, b]$ and the subsequent deaths, possibly after day b, that are a consequence of those infections. We define:

$$\text{IFR}[a, b] = \frac{\text{\# of people infected during } [a, b] \text{ who died}}{\text{\# of infections during the interval } [a, b]}.$$

In this document, we will make use of publicly-available data on the number of daily cases and the number of daily deaths in a range of countries [12] (recall that a *case* denotes a positive test result). We let $\vec{c} = (c_1, \ldots, c_k)$ be the time series of new cases per day for each of the first k days. For our data, day 1 corresponds to March 1, 2020, and day $k = 250$ corresponds to November 6, 2020. Similarly $\vec{d} = (d_1, \ldots, d_k)$ denotes the number of new deaths per day from COVID for each of the first k days. We will also utilize reports of the number of daily tests [14], which we denote by $\vec{t} = (t_1, \ldots, t_k)$. We use $\vec{i} = (i_1, \ldots, i_k)$ to denote our *estimated* number of new infections per day.

4   Estimating the Infections Sequence

In this section, we explain how we determine our estimated sequence of infections: $\vec{i} = (i_1, \ldots, i_k)$. At a high level, we start with the reported number of cases each day: $\vec{c} = (c_1, \ldots, c_k)$. We then incorporate the number of tests each day, $\vec{t} = (t_1, \ldots, t_k)$ and also the results of a one-time antibody test. These three pieces of information give us everything we need.

We will make one simplifying assumption that is needed only for analytical convenience but does not affect the derivation of IFR. Our assumption is that if a person is infected on day j, they either get tested on day j, or never get tested at all. In reality, they might be tested any time after day j, but it will be convenient for us to assume that the testing happens on day j. Note that this assumption will mean that our infections sequence will be slightly shifted forward in time from the true infections sequence. However this will not affect our IFR because, in fitting the infections sequence to the deaths sequence, we still have a "lag" variable that lets us account for an arbitrary time from case to death.

With this simplifying assumption in mind, let us consider an arbitrary day j. Now let's assume we pick a random person on day j. Let I_j be the event that this randomly chosen individual becomes infected on day j. So $\mathbf{P}\{I_j\} = \frac{i_j}{N}$ where N is the population of the country in consideration. Now let T_j be the event that this same randomly chosen individual is tested on day j. So $\mathbf{P}\{T_j\} = \frac{t_j}{N}$. Conditional probability tells us that

$$\mathbf{P}\{I_j\} \cdot \mathbf{P}\{T_j | I_j\} = \mathbf{P}\{T_j \cap I_j\}.$$

Notice that $T_j \cap I_j$ is the event that the randomly chosen individual is both infected and tested on day j – meaning that the individual becomes a "case" on day j (we assume that the test is always accurate). So $\mathbf{P}\{T_j \cap I_j\} = \frac{c_j}{N}$. Putting this all together, we get that

$$\frac{i_j}{N} \cdot \mathbf{P}\{T_j | I_j\} = \frac{c_j}{N}. \tag{1}$$

Thus we can approximate $i_j = \frac{c_j}{\mathbf{P}\{T_j | I_j\}}$ if we know $\mathbf{P}\{T_j | I_j\}$.

Now $\mathbf{P}\{T_j | I_j\}$ represents the fraction of people who are tested, given that they were infected on day j. We will approximate $\mathbf{P}\{T_j | I_j\}$ as being a function

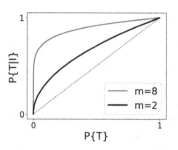

Fig. 2. Red and pink solid curves show our assumed relationship between $\mathbf{P}\{T_j|I_j\}$ and $\mathbf{P}\{T_j\}$, from Eq. 2, for a few values of m. (Color figure online)

of $\mathbf{P}\{T_j\}$, since $\mathbf{P}\{T_j\} = \frac{t_j}{N}$ is a known quantity which should be closely related to $\mathbf{P}\{T_j|I_j\}$. To understand the relationship between $\mathbf{P}\{T_j|I_j\}$ and $\mathbf{P}\{T_j\}$, we first note that infected individuals are more likely to get tested than randomly chosen individuals, since infected individuals may be prompted to get tested by symptoms or contact-tracing. So $\mathbf{P}\{T_j|I_j\} > \mathbf{P}\{T_j\}$. Now consider the ratio between $\mathbf{P}\{T_j|I_j\}$ and $\mathbf{P}\{T_j\}$. This ratio should be highest ($\gg 1$) when $\mathbf{P}\{T_j\}$ is low, because when testing is scarce only people with symptoms will be tested. This ratio should be lowest (converging to 1) when $\mathbf{P}\{T_j\}$ gets high, because at that point, everyone is being tested, regardless of whether they're infected or not.

Figure 2 illustrates a family of possible relationship between $\mathbf{P}\{T_j|I_j\}$ and $\mathbf{P}\{T_j\}$ that satisfies all these intuitions:

$$\mathbf{P}\{T_j|I_j\} = (\mathbf{P}\{T_j\})^{1/m}. \tag{2}$$

We will assume this functional relationship holds for some parameter m, and determine the appropriate m empirically. We tried many possible functions, and found that the family of curves in Eq. 2 yielded the best fit in all of the countries we tried. Thus, via Eq. 1 and Eq. 2, we conclude the following relationship between i_j, c_j, and t_j:

$$i_j = \frac{c_j}{\left(\frac{t_j}{N}\right)^{1/m}}. \tag{3}$$

We will now propose a method for empirically inferring the correct value of $m > 1$. An antibody study tells us, for some day ℓ, the number of people A who were infected prior to day ℓ. Our estimated infections sequence should agree with this figure. Thus we can search for a value of m for which:

$$\sum_{j=1}^{\ell} i_j = \sum_{j=1}^{\ell} \frac{c_j}{\left(\frac{t_j}{N}\right)^{1/m}} \approx A. \tag{4}$$

Notice that $\sum_{j=1}^{\ell} \frac{c_j}{\left(\frac{t_j}{N}\right)^{1/m}}$ is decreasing with respect to m. So, in practice, to find the appropriate value of m, we can do a binary search for m, repeatedly evaluating $\sum_{j=1}^{\ell} \frac{c_j}{\left(\frac{t_j}{N}\right)^{1/m}}$ until Eq. 4 is satisfied.

5 Inferring IFR and Lag Using the Infections Sequence and Deaths Sequence

At this point, we know our estimated sequence of infections $\vec{i} = (i_1, \ldots, i_k)$. In this section, we describe our approach for estimating lag and IFR concurrently.

Our high-level approach is as follows: We assume that the lag time between infections and deaths is a random variable L following a Uniform(a, b) distribution with unknown parameters, a and b, that we will determine.[2] We start with the infections sequence $\vec{i}$. Consider shifting $\vec{i}$ by a particular lag distribution, L, and then vertically scaling the shifted sequence by a particular IFR[3]. The shifted and then scaled sequence is what we call a *candidate death sequence*. We want to choose the candidate death sequence (with its corresponding IFR and L) that best fits the actual death sequence, $\vec{d} = (d_1, \ldots, d_k)$. We return the "best-fit" L and IFR as our final estimate. Part of our process will involve iterating over all possible values for (a, b), assuming some generous upper bound on the lag.

We now explain our approach in more detail. We first define a time shift, $\mathcal{S}_L(\vec{i})$, algorithmically. For each infection in $\vec{i}$, we will sample a new instance ℓ from L and shift the infection forward by ℓ days. This produces a sequence $\mathcal{S}_L(\vec{i}) = (I_1, I_2, I_3, \ldots, I_k)$ where each entry is a random variable denoting the number of shifted infections that fall on that day.

Before we can compare the sequence of random variables, $\mathcal{S}_L(\vec{i})$, to the actual death sequence $\vec{d}$, we need to turn $\mathcal{S}_L(\vec{i})$ into a deterministic sequence, $\bar{\mathcal{S}}_L(\vec{i})$. We define the *unscaled candidate death sequence*, $\bar{\mathcal{S}}_L(\vec{i})$ as

$$\bar{\mathcal{S}}_L(\vec{i}) \equiv (\mathbf{E}[I_1], \mathbf{E}[I_2], \mathbf{E}[I_3], \ldots, \mathbf{E}[I_k]) \equiv (i_1', i_2', i_3', \ldots, i_k'). \qquad (5)$$

To calculate each element i_j' in $\bar{\mathcal{S}}_L(\vec{i})$, we apply linearity of expectations via:

$$i_j' \equiv \mathbf{E}[I_j] = \sum_{w=1}^{j} i_w \cdot \mathbf{P}\{L = j - w\}. \qquad (6)$$

Once we have the deterministic sequence $\bar{\mathcal{S}}_L(\vec{i})$, we will want to compare it to our actual death sequence $\vec{d}$. We define an error metric by $d(\vec{x}, \vec{y}) \equiv \sum_j (x_j - y_j)^2$.

---

[2] We also considered other distributions for lag, such as the LogNormal(μ, σ^2) and Binomial(n, p), but the best results were achieved with the Uniform(a, b).

[3] Although the lag, L, is being applied to the infections sequence $\vec{i}$, the simplifying assumption that we made in Sect. 4 while computing $\vec{i}$ implies that we should think of L as representing a lag between *cases* and deaths.

Given a particular lag distribution L, we now estimate the IFR to be the optimal parameter r which minimizes the error between $r \cdot \bar{S}_L(\vec{i})$ and $\vec{d}$:

$$\text{IFR}_L \equiv \underset{r}{\text{argmin}}\, d\left(r \cdot \bar{S}_L(\vec{i}), \vec{d}\right) = \underset{r}{\text{argmin}} \sum_{j=1}^{k}(r \cdot i'_j - d_j)^2.$$

The right-hand side is quadratic in r and has a unique minimum achieved at

$$\text{IFR}_L = \frac{i'_1 d_1 + \cdots + i'_k d_k}{{i'_1}^2 + \cdots + {i'_k}^2} = \frac{\bar{S}_L(\vec{i}) \cdot \vec{d}}{\left\|\bar{S}_L(\vec{i})\right\|^2}. \tag{7}$$

To find the best candidate death sequence overall, we loop through all choices of the lag distribution, $L \sim \text{Uniform}(a, b)$. We assume any reasonable lag to be well under 50 days, so we restrict $a \leq b \leq 50$. For each pair (a, b), we compute the error given by $d(\text{IFR}_L \cdot \bar{S}_L(\vec{i}), \vec{d})$. We choose the candidate death sequence with the smallest error, and output the IFR and L corresponding to this best candidate death sequence. We describe the entire procedure of estimating L and IFR in Algorithm 5.1.

Algorithm 5.1 BESTFIT$(\vec{i}, \vec{d})$

1:   $M^* \leftarrow \infty,\ a^* \leftarrow \infty,\ b^* \leftarrow \infty,\ r^* \leftarrow \infty$
2:   **for** a in $\{0, \ldots, 50\}$ **do**
3:     **for** b in $\{a, \ldots, 50\}$ **do**
4:       Assume $L \sim \text{Uniform}(a, b)$
5:       Compute $\bar{S}_L(\vec{i})$ via Equations 5 and 6
6:       $r \leftarrow \frac{\bar{S}_L(\vec{i}) \cdot \vec{d}}{\|\bar{S}_L(\vec{i})\|^2}$ // See Equation 7
7:       $M \leftarrow d(r \cdot \bar{S}_L(\vec{i}), \vec{d})$
8:       **if** $M < M^*$ **then**
9:         $M^* \leftarrow M,\ a^* \leftarrow a,\ b^* \leftarrow b,\ r^* \leftarrow r$
10:      **end if**
11:     **end for**
12: **end for**
13: **return** a^*, b^*, r^*

---

6   Inferring IFR in Smaller Time Intervals

Our algorithm thus far assumes that the IFR and lag remain constant throughout the pandemic. In reality, the IFR and lag may change during the pandemic, due to a variety of conditions [4,9]. We will now outline an approach for estimating a time-varying IFR and lag. Throughout our experiments we limit our results to $k = 250$ days, because that is the extent of the data that was available to us at the time of writing this paper.

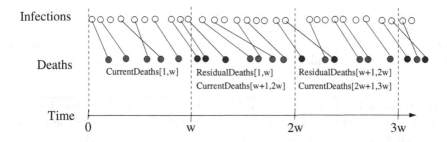

Fig. 3. Time is broken into intervals of length w. For each interval, we show the current deaths in red and the residual deaths from the prior interval in blue. Note that some infections do not result in deaths. Note also that, because the lag is a random variable, the residual deaths and current deaths are sometimes interleaved. (Color figure online)

We refer to our original IFR as IFR$[1, k]$. In this section our goal is to find the best IFR and lag for smaller intervals of length $w < k$, where we imagine that k is a multiple of w. In practice, we will let $w = 50$, because we find that this interval size is small enough to accurately detect changes in IFR without overfitting. We will derive IFR$[1, w]$, IFR$[w + 1, 2w]$, ..., IFR$[k - w + 1, k]$.

Our basic idea is to apply BESTFIT (Algorithm 5.1) to intervals of length w, while accounting for the fact that some deaths may be attributed to infections from the *prior* interval. We call *current deaths of* $[1, w]$ the sequence of deaths which occurred in interval $[1, w]$ that are attributed to infections in $[1, w]$. We define the *residual deaths of* $[1, w]$ as the deaths which occurred after day w but are attributed to infections in $[1, w]$. This terminology is illustrated in Fig. 3. We make the assumption that lag $< w$; thus residual deaths will not span multiple intervals. Therefore, the deaths subsequence, $(d_{w+1}, d_{w+2}, \ldots, d_{2w})$, is the sum of the current deaths of $[w + 1, 2w]$ and the residual deaths of $[1, w]$.

We will compute the residual deaths, IFR, and lag for each interval from left to right. To estimate the residual deaths of $[1, w]$, we first find the best-fit IFR and lag parameters (a^*, b^*) over the interval $[1, w]$, by calculating:

$$(a^*, b^*, \mathrm{IFR}[1, w]) = \textsc{BestFit}((i_1, i_2, \ldots, i_w), (d_1, d_2, \ldots, d_w)), \qquad (8)$$

via Algorithm 5.1. Using the best-fit IFR and lag, we calculate residual deaths of $[1, w]$ by time-shifting and vertically scaling the infections subsequence $(i_1, i_2, \ldots, i_w)$ using a similar construction to $\bar{S}_L(\cdot)$ (see Eq. 5), except that we allow the shifted vector to be longer than the initial vector. For a random variable L with maximum possible value $\ell_{\max}$, we will define the new elongated shift via

$$\bar{S}_L^{\mathrm{long}}(i_1, i_2, \ldots, i_w) \equiv (i'_1, i'_2, \ldots, i'_{w+\ell_{\max}}),$$

where each i'_j is defined as in Eq. 6. Thus to find the residual deaths of $[1, w]$, we compute IFR$[1, w] \cdot \bar{S}_L^{\mathrm{long}}(i_1, i_2, \ldots, i_w)$, where $L \sim \mathrm{Uniform}(a^*, b^*)$, and take all entries after the wth entry.

Moving on to the next interval, we can now find the current deaths of $[w + 1, 2w]$ by subtracting the residual deaths of $[1, w]$ from the deaths subsequence $(d_{w+1}, d_{w+2}, \ldots, d_{2w})$. We then repeat the process of computing residual deaths, IFR, and lag for intervals $[w + 1, 2w], [2w + 1, 3w], \ldots$ (see Algorithm 6.1).

Algorithm 6.1. Computing the IFR in intervals of width w using infections sequence $\vec{i}$ and deaths sequence $\vec{d}$ both of length k. We will use the notation $\vec{v}[s, t]$, for an arbitrary vector $\vec{v}$, to denote $(v_s, v_{s+1}, v_{s+2}, \ldots, v_t)$.

---

curr_l ← 0, curr_r ← w
initialize vector residual_deaths ← $\vec{0}$
while curr_r ≤ k do
   initialize new vector $\vec{d}'$ ← $\vec{d}$[curr_l, curr_r]
   for $1 \leq x \leq \|$residual_deaths$\|$ do
      d'_x ← d'_x − residual_deaths$_x$
   end for
   (a^*, b^*, r^*) ← BESTFIT($\vec{i}$[curr_l, curr_r], $\vec{d}'$)
   Output Uniform(a^*, b^*) and r^* as the best-fit lag and IFR over [curr_l, curr_r]
   Let L denote a random variable distributed Uniform(a^*, b^*)
   residual_deaths ← $r^* \cdot \vec{S}_L^{\mathrm{long}}(\vec{i}$[curr_l, curr_r])[curr_r + 1, curr_r + b^*]
   curr_l ← curr_r + 1, curr_r ← curr_l + w
end while

---

7 Evaluation

In this section, we apply our methodology for determining the IFR and the lag to data for several countries. We make use of 250 days of publicly available data on daily cases and deaths [12] as well as on daily tests [14]. For each country, we will also make use of one antibody study.

United States. In calculating our estimated infections sequence, we assume a population of roughly 382 million [2], 9% of which had been infected by COVID before July 31, 2020 according to the prevalence of antibodies [11]. In Fig. 4(a) we display the raw data. The daily cases sequence, $\vec{c}$, is shown in blue and the daily deaths sequence, $\vec{d}$, is shown in black. In Fig. 4(b) we show the daily tests sequence, $\vec{t}$, in orange. Importantly, the number of daily tests increases a lot over time. In Fig. 4(c) we show our estimated daily infections sequence, $\vec{i}$, in purple (as derived from Eq. 3, where we computed $m = 3.3$ to be optimal). We juxtapose this with our daily cases sequence, $\vec{c}$, shown in blue. *Observe that the purple infection sequence is not simply a vertical scaling of the blue case sequence.* This is because we estimate the daily infections to be a function of *both* the daily cases and daily tests (see Sect. 4), and we can see that the daily tests increase steeply over time (see Fig. 4(b)).

In Fig. 4(d), we apply Algorithm 6.1 with an interval-width of $w = 50$ to our estimated infections sequence from Fig. 4(c) to obtain the best-fit candidate

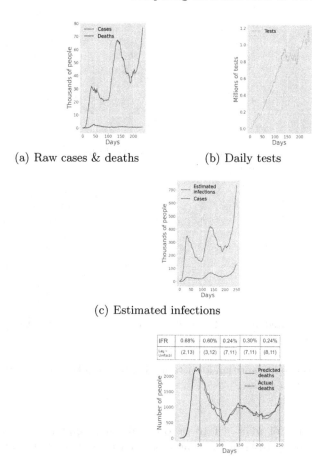

(a) Raw cases & deaths   (b) Daily tests

(c) Estimated infections

(d) Candidate deaths vs. raw deaths sequence

Fig. 4. Illustrating our algorithm for determining IFR and lag for the United States starting March 1, 2020. (Color figure online)

deaths sequence (shown in purple). We juxtapose this with the raw data for deaths, shown in black (same as what we saw in Fig. 4(a), but on different scale). The endpoints of each interval are shown as vertical red lines. Figure 4(d) shows that the IFR decreased over time, eventually changing from 0.68% to 0.24%. Furthermore, the lag is reasonably constant across intervals with the mean lag remaining around 8 days. The best-fit candidate death sequence (purple line) is visually an excellent match to the actual deaths sequence (black line), indicating a low error in our model's optimization. The fact that the lag remains relatively constant across intervals is also an indication that we're not over-fitting.

Italy. We apply our same methodology to Italy (see Fig. 5). We assume a population of roughly 60 million [2], 2.5% of which was infected with COVID before June 20, 2020 according to the prevalence of antibodies [3]. As a result, we

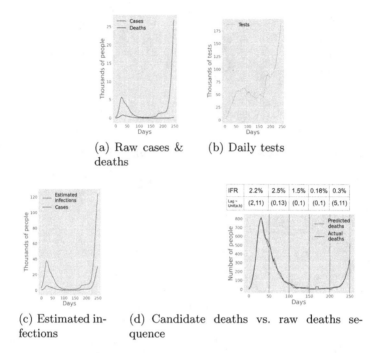

(a) Raw cases & deaths

(b) Daily tests

(c) Estimated infections

(d) Candidate deaths vs. raw deaths sequence

Fig. 5. Illustrating our algorithm for determining IFR and lag for Italy starting March 1, 2020. (Color figure online)

computed a value of $m = 4.1$ to be optimal when applying Eq. 3. As in the United States, daily tests in Italy increase a lot over time. This causes the first peak in infections to make up a larger proportion of the total infections than the first peak in cases makes up in total cases.

Figure 5(d) shows that the IFR in Italy initially increased from 2.2% to 2.5% before dramatically dropping, even reaching as low as 0.18%. The IFR estimates in Italy over the first three intervals are much higher than those of the U.S., which is consistent with news reports that Italian hospitals were overwhelmed during the beginning of the pandemic [6]. Note that the lag was fairly constant with a mean lag around 7 days, except for intervals 3 and 4 which had a lag of almost 0. The unrealistically small lag in these intervals can be attributed to over-fitting, since the deaths graph was essentially flat in these intervals. Time-shifting a flat line doesn't have much of an effect, so the algorithm selected a lag which was fairly arbitrary. Overall, however, the best-fit candidate death sequence (purple line) is visually an excellent match to the actual deaths sequence (black line), indicating that the estimates are generally accurate.

Denmark. In Fig. 6 we show our estimates for Denmark. We assume a population of roughly 5.8 million [2], 1.1% of which had been infected prior to May 15, 2020 according to the prevalence of antibodies [13]. As a result, we computed a value of $m = 4.2$ to be optimal while applying Eq. 3. Figure 6(b) shows that

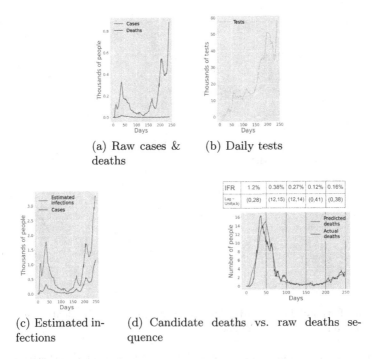

(a) Raw cases & deaths

(b) Daily tests

(c) Estimated infections

(d) Candidate deaths vs. raw deaths sequence

Fig. 6. Illustrating our algorithm for determining IFR and lag for Denmark starting March 1, 2020. (Color figure online)

the daily tests in Denmark rose steadily over time, having a similar effect on the infections sequence compared to the other countries. We estimate that the lag did not change much, with a mean of around 15 days across intervals. The IFR decreased over time changing from 1.2% to 0.38% to 0.27% to 0.12% to 0.16%.

Netherlands. In Fig. 7 we show our calculations for the Netherlands. We assume a population of roughly 17 million [2], 2.8% of which was infected as of April 3, 2020 according to the prevalence of antibodies [23]. As a result, we computed $m = 2.2$ to be optimal in applying Eq. 3. Importantly, we now let day 0 correspond to March 22, 2020 (rather than March 1), since this is when data on daily tests was first reported in the Netherlands [14]. Note that because a small amount of deaths could be attributed to infections that occurred before March 22, 2020, we likely overestimate the IFR in the first interval by a small amount and slightly underestimate the lag (since our model assumes all deaths in the first interval to be attributed to infections in the first interval). As in the other countries, daily tests trended upwards over time, however there was a slight decrease in daily tests towards the end of the pandemic (see Fig. 7(b)). Figure 7(d) shows a visually excellent fit between the predicted deaths sequence and the actual deaths sequence, indicating that our model works well overall. We estimate that the lag stayed relatively constant (with mean of about 7 days), except for a slight increase in the last interval. We estimate that the IFR decreased over

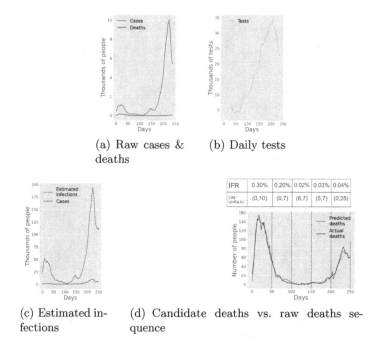

(a) Raw cases & deaths

(b) Daily tests

(c) Estimated infections

(d) Candidate deaths vs. raw deaths sequence

Fig. 7. Illustrating our algorithm for determining IFR and lag for Netherlands starting March 22, 2020. (Color figure online)

time, changing from 0.30% to 0.20% to 0.02% to 0.03% to 0.04%. These IFR estimates are much lower compared to other countries, but follow a similar trend in decrease over time.

8   Conclusions and Future Work

Our approach aims to improve existing IFR estimates via several new ideas. We use data on the daily number of tests to help estimate infections. We treat the lag between cases and deaths as a random variable whose parameters we estimate empirically. We analyze small time intervals, allowing us to estimate a time-varying IFR and lag. In doing so, we find that the IFR in the U.S. decreases over time from 0.68% to 0.24%, with a mean lag between cases and deaths close to 8 days. Our model produces a visually excellent fit to the actual deaths sequence. We also achieve a good fit using data from Italy (IFR decreases from 2.2% to 0.3%), Denmark (IFR decreases from 1.2% to 0.16%), and the Netherlands (IFR decreases from 0.3% to 0.04%).

Overall, our approach for estimating IFR is very different from existing approaches and offers a number of new benefits. We are able to estimate IFR while relying on only a single antibody study, which can be performed at any time. Thus, we can consider an antibody study conducted early on in the pandemic before any individual's antibodies have faded. By contrast, existing approaches may rely on later antibody studies which underestimate the number of infections. Furthermore, our approach readily admits temporal changes. Existing approaches are unable to analyze smaller time-intervals. Lastly, our approach requires few data sources, and in particular doesn't require monitoring individuals. We rely on only a few key reports, each of which was easily accessible from the very start of the pandemic.

There are clearly opportunities for future work on this model. The approach introduced in this paper, for estimating the infections sequence, is novel, and we expect that others will build on this approach to make it more accurate. There is also much work to be done on applying the approach to other countries and regions as more data becomes available.

References

1. Long, Q.X., et al.: Clinical and immunological assessment of asymptomatic SARS-CoV-2 infections. Nat. Med. **26**, 1200–1204 (2020)
2. Countries in the world by population, November 2020. https://www.worldometers.info/world-population/population-by-country/
3. Covid-19, illustrati i risultati dell'indagine di sieroprevalenza (2020). salute.gov.it/portale/nuovocoronavirus/dettaglioNotizieNuovoCoronavirus.jsp?id=4998
4. Data show hospitalized Covid-19 patients are surviving at higher rates, but surge in cases could roll back gains, November 2020. https://www.statnews.com/2020/11/23/hospitalized-covid-19-patients-surviving-at-higher-rates-but-surge-could-roll-back-gains/
5. Estimating mortality from COVID-19, August 2020. https://www.who.int/news-room/commentaries/detail/estimating-mortality-from-covid-19
6. Italy's hospitals overwhelmed by coronavirus as death toll soars (2020). https://www.cbsnews.com/video/italys-hospitals-overwhelmed-by-coronavirus-as-death-toll-soars/
7. Our world in data coronavirus pandemic data explorer, November 2020. https://ourworldindata.org/coronavirus-data-explorer
8. Reasons for a false positive or false negative COVID-19 test result, August 2020. https://www.uchealth.com/en/media-room/videos/reasons-for-a-false-positive-or-false-negative-covid-19-test-result
9. Report of the WHO-China joint mission on coronavirus disease 2019 (COVID-19), February 2020. https://www.who.int/publications/i/item/report-of-the-who-china-joint-mission-on-coronavirus-disease-2019-(covid-19)
10. Daily updates of totals by week and state, February 2021. https://www.cdc.gov/nchs/nvss/vsrr/covid19/index.htm
11. Anand, S., et al.: Prevalence of SARS-CoV-2 antibodies in a large nationwide sample of patients on dialysis in the USA: a cross-sectional study. Lancet Infect. Dis. **369**, 1335–1344 (2020)
12. Dong, E., Du, H., Gardner, L.: An interactive web-based dashboard to track COVID-19 in real time. Lancet Infect. Dis. **20**(5), 533–534 (2020)
13. Espenhain, L., Tribler, S., Jorgensen, C.S., Holm Hansen, C., Wolff Sonksen, U., Ethelberg, S.: Prevalence of SARS-CoV-2 antibodies in Denmark 2020: results from nationwide, population-based sero-epidemiological surveys. https://www.medrxiv.org/content/10.1101/2021.04.07.21254703v1

14. Hasell, J., et al.: A cross-country database of COVID-19 testing. Sci. Data **7**, 1–7 (2020). Article number: 345

15. Levin, A.T., Hanage, W.P., Owusu-Boaitey, N., Cochran, K.B., Walsh, S.P., Meyerowitz-Katz, G.: Assessing the age specificity of infection fatality rates for COVID-19: systematic review, meta-analysis, and public policy implications. Eur. J. Epidemiol. **35**(12), 1123–1138 (2020). https://doi.org/10.1007/s10654-020-00698-1. https://www.medrxiv.org/content/10.1101/2020.07.23.20160895v7

16. Marra, V., Quartin, M.: A Bayesian estimate of the COVID-19 infection fatality rate in Brazil based on a random seroprevalence survey. medRxiv (2020). https://doi.org/10.1101/2020.08.18.20177626. https://www.medrxiv.org/content/early/2020/10/09/2020.08.18.20177626

17. Meyerowitz-Katz, G., Merone, L.: A systematic review and meta-analysis of published research data on COVID-19 infection fatality rates. Int. J. Infect. Dis. Dec. **101**, 138–148 (2020)

18. Newall, A., Leong, R., Nazareno, A., Muscatello, D., Wood, J., Kim, W.: Estimating the infection and case fatality ratio for coronavirus disease (COVID-19) using age-adjusted data from the outbreak on the Diamond Princess cruise ship, February 2020. Int. J. Infect. Dis. Dec. **101**, 306–311 (2020)

19. Padula, W.V.: Why only test symptomatic patients? Consider random screening for COVID-19. Appl. Health Econ. Health Policy **18**(3), 333–334 (2020). https://doi.org/10.1007/s40258-020-00579-4

20. Rossen, L.M., Branum, A.M., Ahmad, F.B., Sutton, P., Anderson, R.N.: Excess deaths associated with COVID-19, by age and race and ethnicity - United States, January 26-October 3, 2020. Morb. Mortal. Wkly Rep. **69**(42), 1522–1527 (2020)

21. Russell, T.W., et al.: Delay-adjusted age- and sex-specific case fatality rates for COVID-19 in South Korea: evolution in the estimated risk of mortality throughout the epidemic. Euro Surveill. **25**(12), 306–311 (2020)

22. Villa, M., Myers, J.F., Turkheimer, F.: COVID-19: Recovering estimates of the infected fatality rate during an ongoing pandemic through partial data (2020). medrxiv.org/content/10.1101/2020.04.10.20060764v1

23. Vos, E.R.A., et al.: Nationwide seroprevalence of SARS-CoV-2 and identification of risk factors in the general population of The Netherlands during the first epidemic wave. J. Epidemiol. Commun. Health **75**(6), 489–495 (2021). https://doi.org/10.1136/jech-2020-215678. https://jech.bmj.com/content/75/6/489

Towards a System to Monitor the Virus's Aerosol-Type Spreading

Guntis Arnicans[1]([✉]) [iD], Laila Niedrite[1] [iD], Darja Solodovnikova[1] [iD], Janis Virbulis[2] [iD], and Janis Zemnickis[1]

[1] Faculty of Computing, University of Latvia, Raina bulvaris 19, Riga 1586, Latvia
guntis.arnicans@lu.lv
[2] Institute of Numerical Modelling, University of Latvia, Riga, Latvia
janis.virbulis@lu.lv

Abstract. Recent scientific studies indicate that attention should be paid to the indoor spread of the Covid-19 virus. It is recommended to reduce the number of visitors to the premises and to provide frequent ventilation of the premises. The problem is that it is not known what the risk of infection is in a particular room at a specific time, when and what actions should be taken to reduce the risk. We offer a system that helps monitor the conditions in the premises with the help of sensors, calculate the risk of infection and provide information to reduce the infection risk. We give an insight into the created prototype with data collection from public spaces and data visualization according to user needs.

Keywords: Indoor air quality · Respiratory infection risk · Covid-19 risk · Sensor data · Visualization · Monitoring system

1 Introduction

Covid-19 has affected people's lives as well as functioning of organizations and countries. Activities to guarantee a secure living and working environment are undertaken. WHO admits that the main way of Covid-19 transmission is through large respiratory droplets. At the same time there are many studies [3,13,20,26] devoted to the Covid-19 transmission through aerosols. The microdroplets, that are smaller than 5 μm, fly beyond 2 m [20] and keep in the air for hours [3], thus calling into question the recommendations of the health authorities. Therefore, the currently recommended protection is not sufficient against the viruses spreading with microdroplets [13]. Researchers recommend different activities to improve the protection, for example, by adequate ventilation [13] or avoiding overcrowding in rooms [21].

Among different technologies used to reduce the impact of Covid-19, Internet of Things (IoT) can be mentioned [4,23]. IoT in healthcare can be used in

---

Supported by the National Research Program of Latvia, Project No. VPP-COVID-2020/1-0025.

Published by Springer Nature Switzerland AG 2021
A. Byrski et al. (Eds.): ANTICOVID 2021, IFIP AICT 616, pp. 95–106, 2021.
https://doi.org/10.1007/978-3-030-86582-5_9

different ways, including for development of efficient epidemic control systems in smart cities or smart buildings [4]. IoT solutions can ensure safe indoor environment by automating ventilation and air-conditioning or by tracking occupant counts [23]. Building management systems with data analysis features are not often used [12], thus a specialized indoor air quality system can be developed. The aspects that can be monitored to reduce Covid-19 transmission in buildings are ventilation and indoor air quality [6]. Besides, relative humidity, temperature, and CO_2 level are named as indicators that can affect infection risk [1].

The paper's authors participated in the project "New Technologies for Targeted Tracing, Testing and Treatment of Covid-19 Patients" (3T) supported by the National Research Program of Latvia. One of the main goals was to trace and proactively prevent in-room spreading of SARS-CoV2 and other respiratory viruses using smart rooms. We propose a solution that uses embedded systems equipped with sensors for the automatic acquisition of indoor parameters. A numerical model describing droplet and aerosol transport physics is developed to assess the risk of virus's spread indoors based on sensor data and multimodal factor analysis. Information about measurements and calculations is visualized and communicated to various users in real-time or for data analysis later. There are many visualization techniques regarding Covid-19 [5]; nevertheless, there are no convenient solutions for indoor monitoring. This paper focuses on sensor data and potential infection risk visualization to reveal weak places in a building and event organizing procedures.

The rest of the paper is organized as follows. Section 2 gives an overview of the model predicting infection risk. Section 3 provides an insight into the architecture of the system implemented during the project and the choice of information visualization means, and Sect. 4 presents an overview of the prototype. Finally, Sect. 5 summarises the achieved results.

2   Infection Risk Modelling

A numerical model for prediction of Covid-19 infection risk was developed within 3T project. The model evaluates the risk of a Covid-19 infection in a particular room based on temperature, humidity, ventilation intensity, the number of people and instances of speech, coughs and sneezing. The virus transport model is integral and mostly uses the mean physical parameter values in the room. Droplets expelled by a potentially infectious person lose mass through evaporation and are partially deposited on the floor. Small particles form an aerosol that can persist for a long time without sedimentation. Virions within the aerosol are transported out of the room via ventilation, partially absorbed by surfaces and lose viability with the time. The droplets and aerosol are inhaled by a person for whom the infection risk is calculated and increasing the infection risk with a time spent in the room. The model is described in detail in [24], the effect of temperature, humidity and ventilation intensity on the infection risk are also demonstrated there. Coughing and especially sneezing greatly increase the probability of infection in the room, therefore, distinguishing these events is crucial.

It is also demonstrated that the model works together with a specially developed dedicated low-cost sensor system [22] which provides all necessary input data for the model.

If the full measurement data set necessary for the model operation is not available, one can measure some of quantities and replace others with typical best guess values. The model can also be used to search for correlations between some conditions in the room and the infection risk. It is obvious that the infection risk is decreased when the concentration of virus containing aerosol in the room is reduced by limiting the number of persons and increasing the ventilation intensity. Increased number of persons and reduced ventilation intensity both raise the CO_2 concentration, which can be measured by commercially available sensors. In this chapter we show how far the infection risk can be correlated with the CO_2 concentration.

The modelled room size is $3 \times 5 \times 3$ m, the temperature is 25 °C, the RH - 50%, both constant. In the first scenario, an infected person enters the room without any virus contamination, stays there for 15 min sneezing once per minute, and leaves the room. After 15 min pause, two healthy persons enter the room and remain there for 15 or 30 min. Cases with different permanent ventilation intensities (30–240 m^3/h) and with/without intensive ventilation of 900 m^3/h (corresponds to open window) during the pause are considered. In the second scenario, the only difference is that one infectious and one healthy person enter the room for the second time.

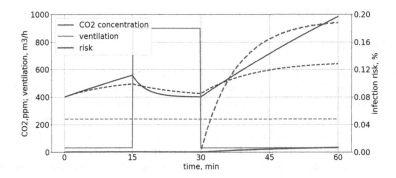

Fig. 1. CO_2 concentration and infection risk vs. time for scenario 1 with permanent ventilation intensity 240 m^3/h (dashed lines) and 30 m^3/h and 900 m^3/h in pause (solid lines)

The CO_2 concentration and the infection risk are shown Fig. 1 for some of the cases as a function of time. In the case with intensive ventilation during the pause (solid lines) the infection risk is considerably smaller. The mean CO_2 concentration during the stay of healthy person in the room and their infection risk at the end of the stay are shown in Fig. 2 for all simulated cases. It can be seen that generally the risk is higher when the CO_2 concentration is higher.

However, the absolute values can differ by orders. The slight decrease of risk at some higher CO_2 concentrations is explained by reduced turbulent mixing and faster sedimentation of small droplets at lower ventilation intensity. The conclusion is that the reduction of CO_2 in room can be used as one measure for the reduction of infection risk, but no recommendations for some CO_2 limit can be given, as it depends also on other parameters.

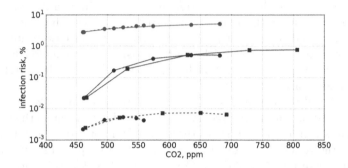

Fig. 2. Infection risk vs. CO_2 concentration for 1st (blue) and 2nd (red) scenarios for 15 min (circles) and 30 min (rectangles) duration of stay; cases with increased ventilation during pause shown with dashed lines (Color figure online)

3   System Design

3.1   Architecture

We developed a solution that included key components to control indoor infection risk in the future during the project. We pay great attention to the presentation of information because a nonspecialist needs to understand the current situation in the premises as quickly and accurately as possible and analyze the indoor environment in the past. The diagram (see Fig. 3) shows only those parts of the system that are essential for risk calculation and provide relevant information for risk management. Other services are not displayed, as their task is to deliver very primitive information about the current situation. If necessary, the specific mobile application required by the room's visitors can be created (during the project, such applications were made).

   Data measurements from the Sensors are received and transferred to the NoSQL database MongoDB. MQTT brokers and MQTT clients connect various devices and services for providing a user with information in real-time, such as Web or mobile applications. All real-time data is stored in the MongoDB database for later data analysis (in fact, other services can work with the data in near real-time). We transfer data to a relational database MySQL. Storing data in a relational database makes it easier to process data, study the data visualization problem, and improve the risk calculation model by using historical data and events from the premises.

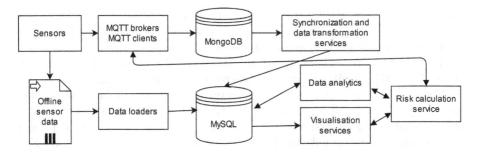

Fig. 3. Conceptual architecture

Some partners have different sensors and their accumulated data. They are not yet connected to the network for operational data transfer. Offline sensor data are received with a delay and are imported into the database with Data loaders. Various visualization experiments are conducted on the data (Visualization services). Besides, data analysis is performed, and new information is added to the database (Data analytics). Risks calculation service calculates the risk of Covid-19 infection in a specific room.

Gradually, we are developing a data model for the necessary data analysis and visualization. Our database stores information about buildings, their premises (rooms) with their characteristics, placed sensors, and their data. Rooms in one building can be connected, and this connection is stored in the form of a plan. It is vital for the project to get information about the number of people in the room, sound events (talking, shouting, coughing, sneezing, etc.), ventilation events (working ventilation system, open windows or doors). The climate in the room is also influenced by the outdoors environment, for which data could also be collected. It is possible to show to building managers the condition of the premises and its changes over time. To survey as much space as possible and obtain data, the sensors change their locations, and the system must ensure proper change management.

3.2   Information Visualisation

For delivery of visual data representation to the end-users in IoT domain usually mobile application or web portal is used, but some authors propose also dashboards [9]. Stephen Few's refined dashboard definition [7] states that "A dashboard is a predominantly visual information display that people use to rapidly monitor current conditions that require a timely response to fulfill a specific role". The dashboard's content should correspond to various requirements of different persons, groups or functions [8] as well as take into account specific needs of its usage domain.

In the IoT domain, an overview is provided [16] that describe chart types and their application rules for specific data sets, as well as tool support for visualization goals. According to analysis purposes, for example, finding a correlation or comparing the data, the best suited chart type should be used [16]. The usage of a particular chart type is determined also by the characteristics of analyzed data [16], for example, how many variables are represented in the data-set.

To understand the existing trends regarding visualization in IoT based indoor air quality (IAQ) monitoring projects, a review of scientific papers was done. We analyzed research papers about IAQ monitoring that were included in another work [18], but we evaluated them from the visualization point of view. We included only such papers, where it was admitted, that the described project provides not only the mobile application but also a web portal. We also analyzed some new research papers including one devoted to the IAQ and Covid-19 [14].

Here we present only concise summary of our findings. The most frequently used are the line charts, but at the same time many sub-types were discovered, whose variations depend on 1) different level of time detail, 2) usage of visual aids, for example, lines representing given maximum level values [25], and 3) how many environmental variables and data sets are depicted on the chart. For example, line chart can represent one variable and two or more data sets for comparison of measurements of different CO_2 sensors in different rooms [17].

There were also other chart types discovered in analyzed papers, but they were used only in few projects. For example, data tables or lists of alerts were used in [11,14]. Map view [10] or widgets [14,27] were used for presenting the real time data. It should be mentioned, that there were also visualizations dedicated for analysis support. Charts from this group demand specific knowledge from the user. For example, cumulative frequency graph [15,17], map of the room [19], box-plots [15], and histograms [2] can be mentioned as a representatives of this visualization type. The user must know the used computation method (e.g., interpolation in [19]) and the charts specification to understand the visualized result.

For our project, we chose to implement a dashboard-type layout of web portal for the user interface. The reports were created according to the purpose of the analysis, the specifics of the data and the user's characteristics, providing an opportunity for timely response according to the visualizations. More sophisticated analytic were also supported for analysis of historical data to reveal regularities. The analyzed experience of other projects in data visualization in the field of IoT was taken into account during the development process of our solution.

4   Prototype

We have placed Aranet4 sensors at the Faculty of Computing of the University of Latvia, Paul Stradins Clinical University Hospital in Covid-19 patients' and doctors rooms, and Riga Teika Secondary School (School). The School's sensors have not yet been connected to our project infrastructure, and we imported offline data about measurements harvested during classes with children.

To verify our approach to providing data according to user needs, we developed a software prototype which supports various visualization and analysis opportunities. The selection of chart types and data represented in them was based on the analysis of techniques used in other projects on IAQ. The reports were built with the aim to present the essential information that may impact Covid-19 distribution and emphasize problem situations in various rooms in a building. To implement the visualization of sensor data in a software prototype we used Grafana for visualization of time series data and Highcharts library to visualize metrics other than time series data. Several report examples follow.

4.1 Initial View

The home page view that is provided in the software prototype (demonstrated in the Fig. 4) is aimed at displaying the operational information about rooms with sensors in buildings. The view shows a plan of several rooms in a building, for instance, rooms at one floor. Sensors are represented as circles positioned in a plan according to their locations in rooms. Circle colors correspond to current values of selected indicators measured by sensors. The ranges of indicator values and their corresponding colors are configured for each indicator. These settings are universal for the whole application and are used in all reports described in the following examples. On the right, the legend explaining the current range settings is shown. Circle colors are automatically refreshed every 10 s to display the newest measurements.

Depending on the analysis objective, a user can choose to display data about a particular indicator, such as CO_2, or alerts that show an indicator with the worse value for each sensor. An indicator along with its value is displayed when a user points on a certain sensor. By looking at the plan view showing alerts, it is possible to observe the overall perspective on the current situation and quickly discover problems in particular rooms.

On the left in the view, the tree of buildings, their plans and rooms, and various reports is shown. It is possible to compare rooms' data from one plan.

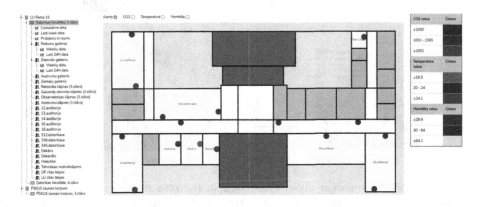

Fig. 4. Fragment of the plan of the Faculty of Computing showing rooms with indicator measurements higher or lower than normal.

4.2   Building Plan Reports

Several types of reports with different visualization techniques are available for each building plan. Such reports allow to compare multiple indicators for several rooms at the same time, detect correlations between their values and analyze differences.

To visualize fluctuations of indicator values measured by sensors installed in several rooms, we utilize line charts shown in the Fig. 5 implemented in Grafana platform. The default time period used for the report is the last week and initially it shows data about all sensors installed in the plan rooms, however, it is possible to change the time period of the report and show/hide lines that correspond to particular sensors. The chart also allows to zoom-in some part of the original time period. The chart demonstrates thresholds defined for indicator values. For example, the low CO_2 concentration is shown in green, however, the high concentration has a red background. In addition to that, working days are displayed with blue background in these charts. Due to space limitations, the chart showing humidity fluctuations is not included in the figure.

The report shown in the Fig. 6 demonstrates the cumulative distribution function (CDF) of CO_2 concentration, temperature and humidity in rooms of a particular building plan during the selected period of time (defaults to the last week). The line charts were implemented with Highcharts library. Thresholds were set according to the same ranges defined for other reports in the application. CDF chart allows to analyze how many times value of a particular indicator exceeded the thresholds during the period. It is also possible to hide/show particular rooms or select types of rooms to be displayed in charts.

To provide analysis of problem situations in rooms within a certain period of time, we created a report shown in the Fig. 7. The report is divided into two parts: one showing recent data for the last week or the last month and another

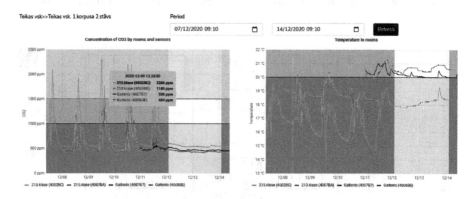

Fig. 5. Weekly information about classrooms in the plan of Riga Teika Secondary School shows fluctuations of CO_2 concentration and temperature where peaks are observed during the classes on working days and low values correspond to beaks between classes and a weekend. (Color figure online)

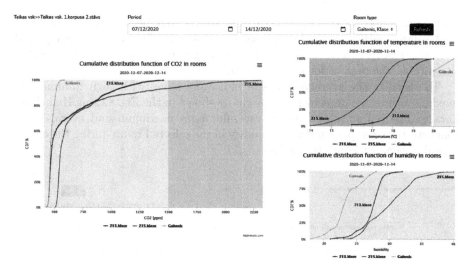

Fig. 6. CDF for selected rooms in the plan of Riga Teika Secondary School allows to compare distribution of indicator values for different room types, for example, hall (shown in green) and classrooms (shown in black and blue). (Color figure online)

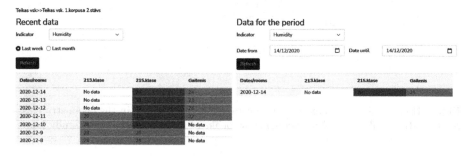

Fig. 7. Healthy and low humidity levels in the hall and classrooms of Riga Teika Secondary School.

allowing to choose any time period. Two parts of the report allow to compare recent indicator values with values in the past. The table in each part of the report includes average indicator values for each room and date. Cell colors are set according to indicator values.

4.3 Room Reports

We have implemented the line charts that show CO_2 concentration, temperature and humidity measured by sensors in a particular room during the last 24 h. Such charts resemble plan charts demonstrated in the Fig. 5, however, they display just one room data. If multiple sensors are installed in the room, the charts show separate lines for each sensor. The points in each line are average values calculated on a 5-min interval. The charts have been implemented utilizing Grafana platform and allow to zoom-in some part of the original time period. It is also possible to select any date period and display data for it to analyze situation in the past or for a longer period.

To visualize the average values of indicators along with their minimal and maximal values, we implemented the charts shown in the Fig. 8 using Highcharts library. The report allows to analyze minimum, maximum and average CO_2 concentration, temperature and humidity in the selected room during the chosen period of time (defaults to the last week).

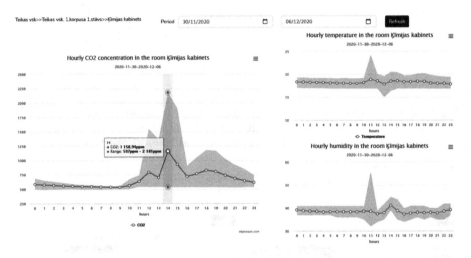

Fig. 8. Hourly minimal, maximal and average indicator values in the chemistry classroom in Riga Teika Secondary School show peaks of all indicators during study hours.

5   Conclusions

During the project, the infrastructure for collecting data from sensors located in public spaces (hospital, university, school) has been created. We have provided an insight into a visualization tool prototype based on research on how to develop the best visualization means aligned with the user's specific demands.

Real-time risk calculation using physical model simulation data is a resource-intensive task that will require a severe computing infrastructure for many thousands of premises. Since the simulation of historical data can be performed, information about typical situations in a room can be obtained. In the case of a school, recommendations were made based on historical data; changes in risk were plotted along with changes in other measurements.

We consulted with various stakeholders with a wide variety of analysis goals and working responsibilities. During the project, it was found that good visualization of data and obtained information is of great importance for the quick reaction according to people's duties if the situation demands and for operational and strategic decision-making as well.

Various organizations, especially educational institutions, are currently actively purchasing sensors for indoor climate control. It is vital to develop the necessary software for effective risk management. The following steps are the systematic evaluation of our prototype by interviewing the end-users from different categories to improve the tool and the proposed visualization means iteratively according to the feedback from the users.

References

1. Ahlawat, A., Wiedensohler, A., Mishra, S.K., et al.: An overview on the role of relative humidity in airborne transmission of SARS-CoV-2 in indoor environments. Aerosol Air Qual. Res. **20**(9), 1856–1861 (2020)
2. Ali, A.S., Coté, C., Heidarinejad, M., Stephens, B.: Elemental: an open-source wireless hardware and software platform for building energy and indoor environmental monitoring and control. Sensors **19**(18), 4017 (2019)
3. Asadi, S., Bouvier, N., Wexler, A.S., Ristenpart, W.D.: The coronavirus pandemic and aerosols: does COVID-19 transmit via expiratory particles? (2020)
4. Chamola, V., Hassija, V., Gupta, V., Guizani, M.: A comprehensive review of the COVID-19 pandemic and the role of IoT, drones, AI, blockchain, and 5G in managing its impact. IEEE Access **8**, 90225–90265 (2020)
5. Comba, J.L.: Data visualization for the understanding of COVID-19. Comput. Sci. Eng. **22**(6), 81–86 (2020)
6. Dietz, L., Horve, P.F., Coil, D.A., Fretz, M., Eisen, J.A., Van Den Wymelenberg, K.: 2019 novel coronavirus (COVID-19) pandemic: built environment considerations to reduce transmission. mSystems **5**(2), e00245-20 (2020)
7. Few, S.: Blog post: there's nothing mere about semantics. https://www.perceptualedge.com/blog/?p=2793. Accessed 14 Apr 2021
8. Few, S.: Information Dashboard Design: The Effective Visual Communication of Data, vol. 2. O'Reilly, Sebastopol (2006)
9. Logre, I., Mosser, S., Collet, P., Riveill, M.: Sensor data visualisation: a composition-based approach to support domain variability. In: Cabot, J., Rubin, J. (eds.) ECMFA 2014. LNCS, vol. 8569, pp. 101–116. Springer, Cham (2014). https://doi.org/10.1007/978-3-319-09195-2_7
10. Marques, G., Miranda, N., Kumar Bhoi, A., Garcia-Zapirain, B., Hamrioui, S., de la Torre Díez, I.: Internet of Things and enhanced living environments: measuring and mapping air quality using cyber-physical systems and mobile computing technologies. Sensors **20**(3), 720 (2020)
11. Marques, G., Roque Ferreira, C., Pitarma, R.: A system based on the Internet of Things for real-time particle monitoring in buildings. Int. J. Environ. Res. Public Health **15**(4), 821 (2018)
12. Minoli, D., Sohraby, K., Occhiogrosso, B.: IoT considerations, requirements, and architectures for smart buildings–energy optimization and next-generation building management systems. IEEE Internet Things J. **4**(1), 269–283 (2017)
13. Morawska, L., Milton, D.K.: It is time to address airborne transmission of coronavirus disease 2019 (COVID-19). Clin. Infect. Dis. **71**(9), 2311–2313 (2020)
14. Mumtaz, R., et al.: Internet of Things (IoT) based indoor air quality sensing and predictive analytic–a COVID-19 perspective. Electronics **10**(2), 184 (2021)

15. Pieš, M., Hájovskỳ, R., Velička, J.: Design, implementation and data analysis of an embedded system for measuring environmental quantities. Sensors **20**(8), 2304 (2020)
16. Protopsaltis, A., Sarigiannidis, P., Margounakis, D., Lytos, A.: Data visualization in Internet of Things: tools, methodologies, and challenges. In: Proceedings of the 15th International Conference on Availability, Reliability and Security, pp. 1–11 (2020)
17. Rinaldi, S., Flammini, A., Tagliabue, L.C., Ciribini, A.L.C.: An IoT framework for the assessment of indoor conditions and estimation of occupancy rates: results from a real case study. Acta Imeko **8**(2), 70–79 (2019)
18. Saini, J., Dutta, M., Marques, G.: Indoor air quality monitoring systems based on Internet of Things: a systematic review. Int. J. Environ. Res. Public Health **17**(14), 4942 (2020)
19. Salman, N., Kemp, A.H., Khan, A., Noakes, C.: Real time wireless sensor network (WSN) based indoor air quality monitoring system. IFAC-PapersOnLine **52**(24), 324–327 (2019)
20. Setti, L., et al.: Airborne transmission route of COVID-19: why 2 meters/6 feet of inter-personal distance could not be enough (2020)
21. Somsen, G.A., van Rijn, C., Kooij, S., Bem, R.A., Bonn, D.: Small droplet aerosols in poorly ventilated spaces and SARS-CoV-2 transmission. Lancet Respir. Med. **8**(7), 658–659 (2020)
22. Telicko, J., Vidulejs, D.D., Jakovics, A.: A monitoring system for evaluation of COVID-19 infection risk. J. Build. Phys. (2021). IOP Conference Series: Materials Science and Engineering (MSE), in press
23. Umair, M., Cheema, M.A., Cheema, O., Li, H., Lu, H.: Impact of COVID-19 on adoption of IoT in different sectors. arXiv preprint arXiv:2101.07196 (2021)
24. Virbulis, J., Sjomkane, M., Surovovs, M., Jakovics, A.: Numerical model for prediction of indoor COVID-19 infection risk based on sensor data. J. Build. Phys. (2021). IOP Conference Series: Materials Science and Engineering (MSE), in press
25. Yang, X., Yang, L., Zhang, J.: A WiFi-enabled indoor air quality monitoring and control system: the design and control experiments. In: 2017 13th IEEE International Conference on Control & Automation (ICCA), pp. 927–932. IEEE (2017)
26. Zhang, R., Li, Y., Zhang, A.L., Wang, Y., Molina, M.J.: Identifying airborne transmission as the dominant route for the spread of COVID-19. Proc. Natl. Acad. Sci. **117**(26), 14857–14863 (2020)
27. Zhao, L., Wu, W., Li, S.: Design and implementation of an IoT-based indoor air quality detector with multiple communication interfaces. IEEE Internet Things J. **6**(6), 9621–9632 (2019)

Comparison Between Two Systems for Forecasting Covid-19 Infected Cases

Tatiana Makarovskikh[ID] and Mostafa Abotaleb[(✉)][ID]

Department of System Programming, South Ural State University,
Chelyabinsk 454080, Russia
Makarovskikh.T.A@susu.ru, abotalebmostafa@bk.ru

Abstract. Building a system to forecast Covid-19 infected cases is of
great importance at the present time, so in this article, we present two
systems to forecast cumulative Covid-19 infected cases. The first system
(DLM-System) is based on deep learning models, which include both
long short-term memory (LSTM), bidirectional long short-term memory
(Bi-LSTM), and Gated recurrent unit (GRU). The second system is a
(TS-System) based on time series models and neural networks, with a
Prioritizer for models and weights for time series models acting as an
ensemble between them. We did a comparison between them in order to
choose the best system to forecast cumulative Covid-19 infected cases,
using the example of 7 countries. As some of them have finished the second wave and others have finished the third wave of infections (Russia,
the United States of America, France, Poland, Turkey, Italy, and Spain).
The criterion for choosing the best model is MAPE. It is a percentage, not an absolute value. It was concluded that an ensemble method
gave the smallest errors compared to the errors of the models in the
(TS-System).

Keywords: Covid-19 · LSTM · BiLSTM · GRU · Deep learning
models · Time series models · ARIMA · BATS · TBATS · Holt's linear
trend · NNAR · Forecasting system

1 Introduction

After more than a year since the spread of the Covid-19 virus in the Chinese
city of Wuhan and its spread around the world, a problem appeared in modeling
and forecasting cases of Covid-19, so there was a need to develop a system that
has the ability to model and predict cases of Covid-19 in addition to obtaining
accurate predictions with the least possible error. At the same time, the scientific
pandemic of Covid-articles began. An enormous number of articles dedicated to

The work was supported by Act 211 Government of the Russian Federation, contract
No. 02.A03.21.0011. The work was supported by the Ministry of Science and Higher
Education of the Russian Federation (government order FENU-2020-0022).

© IFIP International Federation for Information Processing 2021
Published by Springer Nature Switzerland AG 2021
A. Byrski et al. (Eds.): ANTICOVID 2021, IFIP AICT 616, pp. 107–114, 2021.
https://doi.org/10.1007/978-3-030-86582-5_10

different fields dealing with Covid have appeared. Among them, there are thousands of articles devoted to the forecasting of Covid-19 in different countries and regions (especially in South-East Asia and some other countries mostly affected by pandemics). Most of these articles consider one or two models for the fixed data and for the fixed region and look like a news digest. There are two methods for predicting the spread of a pandemic. The first one is based on mathematical models (machine learning, neural networks, time series). The second one is based on data analysis from social media (e.g., tweets, Facebook). For example, In [9] by using a multivariate time series associated with a geographic region, obtained by quantifying indicators from massive online surveys on COVID symptoms, it is offered. Through the Facebook platform, they show how a neural ODE is able to learn the dynamics that connect these variables and detect virus outbreaks in the region. We show that the neural ODE can predict up to sixty days into the future in a virus-spreading environment by analyzing data from US states. Our work focus will be on the mathematical method for forecasting cumulative daily Covid-19 infection cases.

In our article, we consider two forecasting systems that allow us to choose the best model to analyse the time series appearing as input data. The first system (DLM-system) is based on deep learning models that include LSTM, BiLSTM, and GRU. The second system (TS-system) is based on time series and neural network models, which include models (NNAR, BATS, TBATS, Holt Linear trend, and ARIMA). We also designed a weight-through Prioritizer for models and gave weights where it assigns weights to the time series models and neural network model and gets the Ensembling model and compares its errors with the errors of each model of time series and neural networks in the second system (TS-system), where the Ensembling model very accurate results were given in five countries (Russian federation - France - Poland - Turkey - Italy) out of seven countries (Russia, the United States of America, France, Poland, Turkey, Italy, and Spain). As some of them have finished the second wave and others have finished the third wave of infections. The Prioritizer idea is due to giving a higher weight to the best model and the remaining models give it constant weights. In [1] It is shown that Holt's linear trend model is better than the ARIMA model for China, Italy, and the USA. In [4] used RNN, LSTM, (SARIMA) Seasonal Autoregressive Integrated Moving Average, and Holt winter's exponential smoothing and moving average methods to forecast Covid-19 cases in Iran. Their comparative study on these methods showed that the LSTM model outperformed other models in terms of the least error values for infection development in Iran. In [8] We concluded that it is difficult to obtain a highly accurate forecast without periodically updating the model's parameters. As a result, the development of a system to automatically select the best forecasting model and its best parameters is critical. In [10] Models ranked from good performance to the lowest in all scenarios are Bi-LSTM, LSTM, GRU, SVR, and ARIMA. Bi-LSTM generates the lowest MAE and RMSE values of 0.0070 and 0.0077, respectively, for deaths in China. The best R squared score value is 0.9997 for recovered cases in China. On the basis of demonstrated robustness and enhanced prediction accuracy, Bi-LSTM can be exploited for pandemic prediction.

Given the similarity in the characteristics of the models in the United States and Italy, it was suggested that in [11] that the corresponding forecasting tools can be applied to other countries facing the Covid-19 pandemic, as well as to any pandemics that may arise in the future. However, a general principle for choosing models for forecasting the spread of Covid-19 has not yet been formulated. Moreover, for different states and different conditions for the spread of the epidemic, it is advisable to build a forecast using different models. For example, in [6]. The LSTM model was shown that had consistently the lowest rates of forecast errors for tracking the dynamics of infection cases in the four countries considered. There are also studies that show that the ARIMA model and cubic smoothing spline models had lower forecast errors and narrower forecast intervals compared to Holt's and TBATS models.

As for the SIR model, even at the beginning of the pandemic, it was shown to be ineffective in predicting cases of coronavirus infection. For example, using this model, it was found that the peak of the second wave of infection cases in Pakistan should have occurred on August 25, 2020. However, in fact, the peak of infections in this country was in December 2020 [7]. The "covid19.analytics" package, developed by using the R language for programming, has the same drawbacks. This is evidenced by the results of the SIR model and the prediction of the time of occurrence of the second (and subsequent) wave cycles. Because of these drawbacks to epidemiological models in dealing with Covid-19, there was a need to rely on time series models and deep learning models for their accuracy in detecting the pattern of the spread of Covid-19 and predicting cases of infection. As a result, two systems were created: one that relies on deep learning models and the other that relies on time series and neural network models and combines them and gives weights to time series models through the Prioritizer.

2   The Review of Two System for Forecasting Covid-19

The purpose of our work is to create an algorithm that allows for the available initial data on the spread of coronavirus infection in a certain region for a given period of time to determine the best model for making a forecast for a given period. The algorithm analyses forecasts from time series models (TS-system) (ARIMA, Holt's linear model, BATS, and TBATS), and the neural networks model (NNAR) and selects a model that produces a forecast with a minimum mean absolute percentage error (MAPE). The article describes a R program (TS-system) that generates a forecast using the above-mentioned models and combines them with them and weights for each time series model using the Prioritizer. On the other hand, we apply (DLM-system) deep learning model systems and compare both systems' errors to obtain accurate forecasts with the least MAPE errors.

Figure 1 shows global variables for running the second system (TS-system) that is based on time series models and a neural network model.

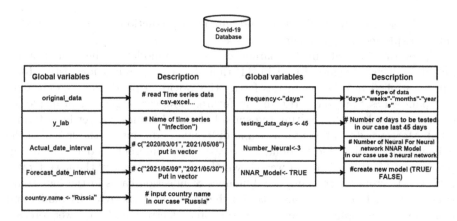

Fig. 1. Global variables for running the second system (TS-system) that is based on time series models and a neural network model.

Figure 2 It shows the scheme of the developed second system (DLM-system), which allows us to choose the best model with the available initial data.

This software module works according to the following algorithm.

Figure 3 shows the idea of the Prioritizer for models and giving weights, where after obtaining expectations from the time-series models and neural networks, they are Ensembling and given weights. It was found that giving a weight of 0.9 to the best model of the time series and neural networks, and distributing (1–0.9) equally over the other models gives accurate results and fewer errors.

Algorithm Covid-19 Forecasting

Step 1. Insert time series data, Covid-19, and global variables (see Fig. 2).

Step 2. Split the data into training and testing.

Step 3. Transform time series to be stationary, and supervised. Using the first system (DLM-system) for deep learning models.

Step 4. Run deep learning models by using the first system (DLM-system).

Step 5. Using the second system, (TS-system) we run time series models and neural Network (NNAR) model, and ensembling them between them using a prioritizer for models and giving weights for each model.

Step 6. Calculate the accuracy of the training data (ME-MAE-RMSE-MPE-MAPE-MASE-ACF).

Step 7. Calculate the accuracy of the testing data (MAPE), and obtain the summary tables for forecasting by using each model for each system (DLM-system and TS-system).

Step 8. Select the best model for forecasting with the least error MAPE.

The source code for two systems for forecasting Covid-19 using this algorithm is published on GitHub [3].

The TS-system selects the best model from five time-series models forecasting Covid-19 with the least error in the MAPE. Note that the considered system

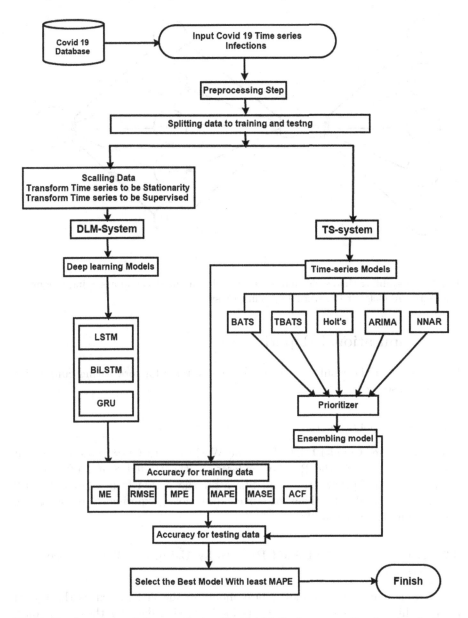

Fig. 2. For forecasting daily cumulative Covid-19 infection cases, the structural scheme consists of two systems (DLM-system and TS-system).

can be used to forecast not only the time series associated with the spread of the epidemic. The study of this system implementation for other time series (for example, to forecast the production volume, the prices of goods, etc.) is a topic for further research.

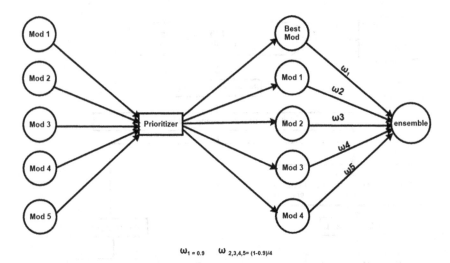

$\omega_{1} = 0.9$ $\omega_{2,3,4,5} = (1-0.9)/4$

Fig. 3. Ensembling time series models by prioritizing models and assigning weights to time series models for the second system (TS-system).

3   Computational Experiments

Let us consider the results of using the two systems for forecasting cumulative infection cases [2].

3.1   Covid-19 Datasets

The system uses Covid-19 data from the World Health Organization [5] about Covid-19 infection in the Russian Federation, the United States of America, France, Poland, Turkey, Italy, and Spain for the period from March, 1, 2020 to May, 8, 2021. We use them for our computational experiments by using two systems, the following in [2]:

3.2   Analysing the Obtained Results by Using the Two Different Systems

From Table 1, it is clear that the best model in the first system is the LSTM model, which achieved the least errors in the testing data for the last 45 days in all seven countries. We can see that the LSTM model is the best one for forecasting cumulative daily Covid-19 infection cases.

From Table 2, it is clear that the best model in the (TS-system) is the Ensembling model, which achieved the least errors in the testing data for the last 45 days in five countries. We can see that the Ensembling model is the best one for forecasting cumulative daily Covid-19 infection cases.

Table 3, shows the subdivision of the considered countries into two groups according to the best forecasting system used (DLM-system and TS-system).

Table 1. MAPE % for Model selection for forecasting cumulative daily Covid-19 infection cases by using the (DLM-system) Deep learning system.

Country	LSTM	BiLSTM	GRU	Best model
Russian federation	0.042257	0.094228	3.634369	LSTM
USA	1.037883	1.23026	1.622161	LSTM
France	0.231087	3.588404	2.273541	LSTM
Poland	1.324627	7.303683	6.399338	LSTM
Turkey	3.117724	4.556783	21.827662	LSTM
Italy	0.246362	2.550975	7.110975	LSTM
Spain	0.888655	1.558458	8.811285	LSTM

Table 2. MAPE % for Model selection for forecasting cumulative daily Covid-19 infection cases by using the (TS-system) time series models and the neural Network (NNAR) model.

Country	NNAR	BATS	TBATS	Holt's	ARIMA	ARIMA model	Ensembling	Best model
Russia	2.766	0.071	0.079	0.099	0.316	ARIMA(1, 2, 4)	0.018	Ensembling
USA	3.465	0.627	0.633	0.612	0.795	ARIMA(3, 2, 2)	0.689	Holt model
France	9.37	2.291	2.32	1.229	0.909	ARIMA(2, 2, 3)	0.825	Ensembling
Poland	2.897	3.462	3.43	5.188	4.194	ARIMA(3, 2, 2)	2.305	Ensembling
Turkey	1.793	9.036	9.094	8.986	9.334	ARIMA(2, 2, 2)	1.402	Ensembling
Italy	3.265	3.897	2.021	2.37	3.066	ARIMA(2, 2, 2)	1.969	Ensembling
Spain	5.651	2.007	1.439	0.746	1.355	ARIMA(5, 2, 0)	0.931	Holt model

Table 3. MAPE % for System selection for forecasting cumulative daily Covid-19 infection cases.

Country	Least error for the (DLM-system)	Least error for the (TS-system)	Best system
Russian federation	0.042257	0.018	TS-system
USA	1.037883	0.612	TS-system
France	0.2310873	0.825	DLM-system
Poland	1.324627	2.305	DLM-system
Turkey	3.117724	1.402	TS-system
Italy	0.246362	1.969	DLM-system
Spain	0.888655	0.746	TS-system

4 Conclusion

So, we compared the (TS-system) with (DLM-system) deep learning models (LSTM-BI-LSTM-GRU) and compared their errors. When comparing (DLM-system) models' errors and Ensembling model errors, it was found that Ensembling models yielded fewer errors at the level of 4 countries, so we found that the second system was able to outperform (DLM-system) deep learning models at the level of four countries through Ensembling between them by using a Prioritizer for models and giving weights for time series that were added in the second system. Thus, we conclude that expectations can be obtained. By Ensembling models in the (TS-system), errors can be reduced.

The open task is testing the (TS-system) for epidemic data for different countries and different ways of Covid-19 infections spreading to get the low MAPE forecasting of infection cases and to define the optimal criteria for choosing the best model.

References

1. Abotaleb, M.S.A.: Predicting COVID-19 cases using some statistical models: an application to the cases reported in China Italy and USA. Acad. J. Appl. Math. Sci. **6**(4), 32–40 (2020)
2. Abotaleb, M., Makarovskikh, T.: Comparison between two systems for forecasting COVID 19 cumulative infected case (2021). https://rpubs.com/abotalebmostafa/771031
3. Abotaleb, M., Makarovskikh, T.: Two systems for forecasting COVID-19 (2021). https://github.com/abotalebmostafa11/2-systems-for-forecasting-covid-19
4. Azarafza, M., Azarafza, M., Tanha, J.: COVID-19 infection forecasting based on deep learning in Iran. medRxiv (2020)
5. Our World in Data: Daily COVID 19 vaccine doses administrated (2021). https://ourworldindata.org/grapher/daily-covid-19-vaccination-doses
6. Gecili, E., Ziady, A., Szczesniak, R.D.: Forecasting COVID-19 confirmed cases, deaths and recoveries: revisiting established time series modeling through novel applications for the USA and Italy. PLoS ONE **16**(1), e0244173 (2021)
7. Hussain, N., Li, B.: Using R-studio to examine the COVID-19 patients in Pakistan implementation of sir model on cases. Int. J. Sci. Res. Multidisc. Stud. **6**(8), 54–59 (2020)
8. Makarovskikh, T.A., Abotaleb, M.S.: Automatic selection of ARIMA model parameters to forecast Covid-19 infection and death cases. Vestnik Yuzhno-Ural'skogo Gosudarstvennogo Universiteta. Seriya Vychislitelnaya Matematika i Informatika **10**(2), 20–37 (2021)
9. Núñez, M., Barreiro, N., Barrio, R., Rackauckas, C.: Forecasting virus outbreaks with social media data via neural ordinary differential equations. MedRxiv (2021)
10. Shahid, F., Zameer, A., Muneeb, M.: Predictions for COVID-19 with deep learning models of LSTM. GRU and Bi-LSTM. Chaos Solitons Fractals **140**, 110212 (2020)
11. Tian, Y., Luthra, I., Zhang, X.: Forecasting COVID-19 cases using machine learning models. MedRxiv (2020)

A Pandemic Digital Global Architecture

Maurice J. Perks$^{(\boxtimes)}$

Todber, UK

Abstract. This paper is a proposal for a global IT health system. As a paper, it is concerned with the high-level definition of the architecture of such a system. If designed and deployed correctly, a system that will be of benefit to the world when faced with a pandemic. Therefore, this paper is not written in the style of a scientific research document with details about findings and conclusions. Instead, its focus is on proposing an architectural model and the beginning of designing and implementing a Global Health IT System that can benefit everyone.

It is a paper that is focused on concepts and does not discuss in-depth detail. How-ever, that detail is undoubtedly considerable and necessary as the proposed system development and deployment proceeds.

This paper defines a model for politicians, social specialists, medical experts, and IT computer science experts. A model they can have in their minds to begin a significant change to how risk can be managed. A change to how our global society acts and reacts when faced with the threat of a pandemic.

This paper aims to inform key international decision-makers that Computer Science can play a significant part in controlling a pandemic. And begin the definition of the system solution to do this. This paper is a signpost to what must be done.

Keywords: Pandemic digital global architecture · Pandemic Dashboard Information System (PDIS) · Pandemic status · Pandemic outcome · Global health system

1 Introduction

The Covid-19 pandemic has shaken the foundations of societies everywhere. It is a major medical, economic, and social challenge. It is also a Computer Science challenge; how Information Technologies (IT) can provide insight into the pandemic's state. Examples of such a system can be found in [3,4]. These IT systems are global, and transaction driven and are examples of how IT systems can operate instantaneously and continuously.

Today, IT systems are essential in dealing with the pandemic through appropriate medical and social actions. The success of these systems is critical.

M. J. Perks—Independent IT Consultant, Retired IBM Fellow, FBCS.

The preparedness of nations to have IT systems ready for execution was not ideal when the Covid-19 pandemic appeared. Time to react to a pandemic is key in dealing with it efficiently. This paper assumes components of the IT system proposed, whether hardware, software, or skills, can be brought together by the disciplines of Computer Science into a real-time operational system. What is needed is the realisation of the need for such systems and the political, social, and financial push to meet the challenge. In short: **we have the technology; we need the sponsorship.**

2   Background on Readiness

In dealing with the Covid-19 pandemic, the UK had many IT systems collecting, analysing, and reporting on the pandemic's state. The UK is used as an example; other nations may have better or worse systems that they employed. There is no global system, thereby no global focus on what is happening.

During the start of the Covid-19 pandemic, there was a time lag in collecting and analysing the critical data needed to take swift and corrective decisions to control its progress. There was confusion about what the data told the medical experts and the politicians. Information was inaccurate, late, and came from too many sources. One of the most annoying and sometimes dangerous outputs of IT information systems is misinformation.

The technology components for an effective IT system, the hardware and many software components were available. The overall system and the processes to execute them were not. Over time a potpourri of systems was refined into one apparent system with consistent inputs and outputs. Time was lost, and actions derived from the information available were not optimised. Thereby solutions were not optimised.

3   What Is Needed?

3.1   Status and Outcome Trusted Information

When a pandemic is or is about to happen to a region, precise information is needed with various degrees of granularity. There are two key questions to answer:

1. Where are we with the pandemic?
   - The Current Status. What is happening, and at what stage of the pandemic are we today?
2. Where are we going with the pandemic?
   - The Possible Outcomes. Where will we be within a prescribed timeframe like days, weeks, months?

With timely and accurate answers, medical and social containment measures can be determined and put into action. However, the answers to crucial questions need to be produced in real-time to achieve maximum effect. Any timeliness lag of information means a lag in the effectiveness of the measures to combat the pandemic. The ultimate design point of a pandemic digital system must therefore be real-time. When any pertinent event occurs, the relevant data is collected, analysed, and the derived information reported. This is probably a goal that cannot be achieved in the early life of the system, but any variance from real-time must be as small as possible.

Of particular focus is the rate of transmission of a virus. A pandemic can spread very quickly, locally, or globally. For example, the Covid-19 pandemic was generally identified in Hunan, China, in late 2019. Some two months later, the virus was global. In the UK, what is known as the English variant was identified in September 2020. It spread throughout the UK and many other countries within weeks with a surprising speed after the experiences of other variants. For references illustrating that there is a time before a variant is detected, but very quickly it is transmitted see [2, 9].

The message is that a pandemic can spread and snowball very rapidly. So, the IT system described here to deal with a coming pandemic must be architected to collect input data and output information in real-time. We can, for this paper, entitle such a system as:

The Pandemic Dashboard Information System (PDIS)

3.2   The Skills Needed

From the outset, it must be realised that considerable and varied skills will be needed to create and operate a PDIS. Essential skills are shown in Fig. 1.

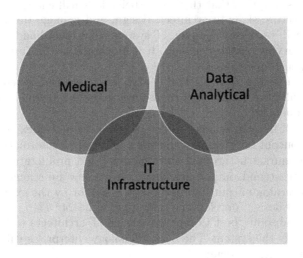

Fig. 1. The skill set

Without the correct mix of these skills, the appropriate system will not be of value.

- Medical skills to define the requirements of what must be collected, analysed, and in particular reported. The experts possessing these skills know what they want.
    - Where are we with the pandemic?
        * What has happened? When did it start and how did it grow?
        * What is happening? How is it growing within regions and between regions?
    - Where are we going with the pandemic?
        * What could happen? What course could it take from today?
        * Is it spreading like a past pandemic, or is its spreading in a novel way? What patterns can we see and extrapolate?
- Data Analytical skills to define the base data and how it will be analysed for the medical experts. There will be a need for analysis tools, including Artificial Intelligence (AI). The system must learn and improve.
    - What programming functions do we need to transform the data into information?
        * What tools do we have to be able to provide the crucial information to the medical and social experts?
    - What mathematics do we need in the analysis programming?
        * The most suitable mathematics must be chosen. The choice will need exceptional skills. Simple extrapolations based upon base assumptions will not be sufficient.
        * There must be a consideration of the Dynamic Complexity of the problem to be solved and associated mathematics [10]. The assumption must be that new pandemics may not behave like past pandemics. Even when the behaviour of a pandemic is understood, there must be an assumption that the known behaviour will change.
- IT Infrastructure skills to architect, design, and manage the infrastructure. The PDIS will be a very complex IT system. that must handle sudden input peaks and varying output demands. It will operate 24 * 7. Key challenges will come from such questions as:
    - How do I design, develop, and deploy, in phases, the system?
        * It will have hundreds of thousands, perhaps millions upon millions of components.
        * It will have to handle sudden input peaks and unexpected demands for output information, what we might call an Information Pandemic.
        * The infrastructure will start minimal and proliferate as new points of input and output are added. And, new functionality, especially concerning output information, is asked for by the experts.
    - How do I design, develop and operate it to be 24 * 7?
        * The absolute best Computer Science IT architects will be needed to specify the system. The best technology enterprises will supply these along with academia.
        * There will be considerable component redundancy.

4 The Pandemic Dashboard Information System (PDIS)

4.1 The Purpose of the PDIS

The purpose of the PDIS is to provide information to a nation's medical, social, and political factions, a group of nations and especially the international scene when a pandemic threatens and is becoming global.

The foundation or basic Architectural Building Blocks of the PDIS are Data, Information, and Infrastructure, as shown in Fig. 2 below. Data is collected and stored by the system and transformed by analysis into information. For example, experts require information to understand how the pandemic in question progresses and can be controlled.

The infrastructure hosts and operates the system; it is, therefore, a shared international infrastructure with some central nodes like server farms and datastores in centres and many, many distributed nodes. In the extreme, in some years' time, the endpoints could even be microchips, or their descendants, attached to people so that their individual states like positive or negative concerning infection can be monitored instantly. There will be two operational phases.

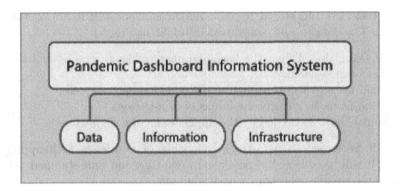

Fig. 2. The basic building blocks

4.2 Operational Phase 1. Regular Monitoring and Predicting

This will be the normal state of the PDIS when it runs in silent mode. The system observes the global scene where viruses have been reported and are becoming candidates for a pandemic. The system predicts how a local outbreak might spread to become a major pandemic. Prediction is based on known, experienced before patterns and advanced mathematical analysis of unseen and unknown patterns, probable and improbable patterns. Complex predictive analysis methods having generated such patterns[1].

---

[1] Prediction is very difficult, especially if it's about the future! Niels Bohr, Nobel Laureate.

The Key Questions to be answered are:

- Where are we with the pandemic?
- Where are we going with the pandemic?

4.3   Operational Phase 2. Pandemic Reporting

This will be an operational phase when a nation or region is close to declaring a pandemic or is subjected to a pandemic state. There will be four main activities:

1. Collection of data from specific areas.
2. Standard Analysis, based upon routine reporting of base metrics.
3. Special Analysis, as required by experts to investigate special conditions.
4. Reporting, to experts.

The PDIS will predict how a possible pandemic will behave over time. A model for this type of operational analysis may be weather forecasting (cf. [7]).

4.4   Data

Data is collected and stored by the system, and parts of it are continuously analysed. The data can be categorised into four main sets:

1. Static Data, that defines the basic parameters like geography and the basic metrics of the system.
2. Personal Data, which is enough to define individual cases etc.
3. Infection Data, to identify the intensity of infections.
4. Technical Data, as needed by the applications of the system.

Data will be stored in datastores consisting of databases with appropriate indexes. It will be collected, if possible, in real-time and time-stamped. All data will be duplicated synchronously as a minimum.

A complex data analysis engine is at the heart of the PDIS, and its components are analysis tools. All data, when transmitted or stored, will conform to accepted international standards. Some tasks will have consistent execution profiles that will not change. Others will be ad-hoc tasks.

Data collection endpoints should include individual personal devices, testing facility systems, medical systems, vaccination facilities.

Data and associated information on past patterns of a pandemic will also be needed for projected outcomes. Still, there will always be some unexpected or never-before-seen outcomes as happened with the Covid-19 pandemic. Historical data will be analysed and reanalysed to reveal unknown information and patterns that we not detected previously. Academic programs and projects will be ideal for this set of tasks.

All data elements, particular personal case data, will be held securely and not open to general/public access. Data will be depersonalised wherever this is possible.

4.5   Information

The information produced by the PDIS will be of two types:

- Standard Regular Continuous Information, which is as close as possible to real-time information. It has been predecided as being the core information that the PDIS will produce and output. This information will be provided continuously or at regular predetermined intervals.
- Ad-hoc Irregular Information is to answer specific queries resulting from requests by experts to abstract particular information pertinent to their view and assessment of the pandemic. Such information will require advanced analysis tools and a close working relationship between medical/social experts and analysis experts.

4.6   Infrastructure

The infrastructure will have internationally distributed components that collect and assemble data and central components that store and analyse data. There must be no single point of failure of the total system. Some components will be owned and operated nationally, and some will be under international control.

All interfaces within the system will be defined and prescribed through standards. Where standards for data formats already exist, these will be used. Where they do not they will be specified and mandated. In addition, all interfaces will be secure to prevent unauthorised data extraction or malicious activities on the system.

Standard network Internet protocols and transport channels will be used. Special high-throughput data pipes will connect the main centres. The encryption of data will be standard.

5   Key Design Points

5.1   Timeliness

The assumption is that a virus can spread rapidly. The Covid-19 pandemic has shown that variants appear and spread more rapidly than their predecessors. The designation of a pandemic is a social-political decision based upon expert medical advice. It is not an IT decision. A central design point of the PDIS is that it must report in real-time or near real-time (say within minutes). Thereby a pandemic can be immediately declared after it is initially detected. It can then monitored and measured.

The PDIS is a health warning system and must be seen as an Early Warning System. A system that reduces the risks inherent in disasters by quickly providing information, so there is time for preventative actions (see e.g. [11]).

5.2   Ownership, Sponsorship, and Funding

A PDIS should be a national function and be part of a national or region's Risk Management. There are many examples of national risk management systems (see, e.g. [6]). Each nation or region has to decide how the system is funded. In addition, the PDIS must be seen as an international system and be formally supported. For example, it might be sponsored by The World Health Organization (WHO) [8].

The PDIS should be an essential national or regional asset. It must be part of the nation's prime Risk Management, The Pandemic Risk Management component. Unless such a discipline originating from a system like the PDIS is part of both international and national risk management, the recurrence of another pandemic after the Covid-19 pandemic could bring about similar or worse social and economic effects.

In the section of this paper, The High-Level PDIS Architecture Model—The Physical Components, which follows reference is made to existing global financial system models [1,5]. The Business Model for these systems is based upon them being user-financed. The PDIS will, of course, be politically/socially financed.

Unless the population sees the need for the PDIS and trusts the system's continuous data collection, and output information, it will not succeed. Without formal international recognition, there will be no global pandemic single system image. Instead, each new pandemic will be treated as a surprise like the Covid-19 pandemic has been.

6   The High-Level PDIS Architecture Model

6.1   Functional Components

The PDIS will have the following Functional Components. The interrelationship of these is shown in Fig. 3.

1. Data, and its collection and storage.
2. Execution Mode, the running state in which the data is analysed.
3. Information, outputs that guide the experts and warn of a potential pandemic and the state of an existing pandemic.
4. Infrastructure, on which the system executes.
5. Skill Sets, by which the system is designed, deployed, and operates and is continuously improved.
6. Sponsorship, by which the system is created, funded and controlled.

The system components, wherever possible, will work in a synchronised real-time mode. Input data will be processed as a series of transactions that events have generated. As many current states of the pandemic as possible will be analysed in real-time or near real-time. Information will also be generated and presented as near as possible in real-time.

There will be a set of preset triggers. Then, when one or more of these are exceeded or receded, this can be reported to those experts responsible for medical and social decisions. So, that a pandemic can be declared – it's going to happen, or undeclared – it is not going to happen, or it's over.

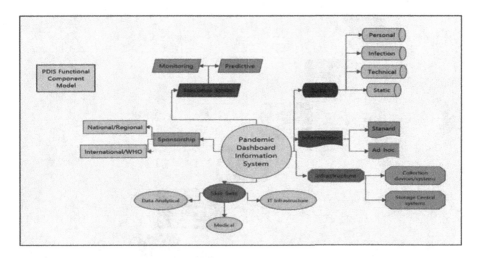

Fig. 3. The functional components of the PDIS

6.2   The Physical Model

The physical model of the PDIS will be a set of interlinked IT node systems that exchange data and information about the pandemic and how its state is changing. Queues will inevitably form at some sub-system nodes. The overall model is like a global credit card system or a global payments system (for examples of real-time global financial systems see [1,5]). The financial world has long exploited and refined such IT models with 24 * 7 operations, high security and instant responses to requests and data transmission. Some of these systems have existed for 50 years or more and prove that the likes of the PDIS real-time system can be built and successfully run.

7   Key Decisions

A set of primary and Key Decisions must be made to begin and then get the PDIS into operation.

The PDIS will evolve as a global operational system. It will not suddenly happen but must not take to years to begin to happen. It must have a phased implementation to provide some benefits reasonably short, say three years. A long project that does not deliver early benefits will soon lose sight of the goal. The goal is to reduce the risk of a new pandemic. The first version will be limited regarding the data it collects, the analysis it does and the information it provides. But it must make the earliest possible contributions to the social and medical challenge of dealing with a global pandemic.

The following high-level chart (see Fig. 4) shows the Key Decisions and activities that must be made. These involve political, social, medical and computer science participants.

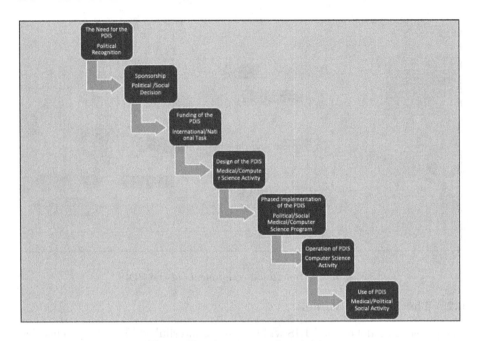

Fig. 4. Key decisions and activities

A fundamental assumption is that there is political and social willpower to have the PDIS for the international benefits. This must be proven and transcribed into a program to deliver the PDIS.

Plus, there is an assumption that medical and computer science expertise is needed to design and develop it and make it work. This paper states as a basic tenet that Computer Science expertise does exist if applied to the task with rigour. So do the IT components.

8   Conclusion and Proposal

The speed at which the Covid-19 pandemic grew caught the world by surprise. In the middle of 2021, there is still a degree of surprise on how the same pandemic regrows in waves.

Computer Science played a vital part in how the pandemic was, and is, measured, reported, and actioned. However, specific and focused IT systems were slow to become operational. Often giving inaccurate outputs and a fragmented view of the pandemic both globally and regionally. The PDIS is a proposed architecture for what we can call an international Pandemic Defense system and a set of national Pandemic Defense systems that are up and running in time for the next potential pandemic.

The world must have an operational system that can measure and predict the risks of a pandemic growing and happening. If a pandemic does occur, the PDIS is an up-to-date instrument, a social tool,

that measures and informs of a pandemic's progress in near real-time. Without the creation of PDIS's the world will again be slow to use both the skills and components of IT to measure the degree of a pandemic's challenge. The use of IT will be fragmented. At the start of the 21st century, we have the components to design and deploy the system. There is a singular message:

Computer Science has the technology; we need the sponsorship.

Finally, it's interesting to reflect that had the Covid-19 virus appeared in, say, 2010[2], it would have taken years for appropriate vaccines to have been developed. Vaccines capable of combating the virus.

In 2020 it took months because the medical world was prepared. The vaccine research world was ready, but the global pandemic information system was not in place. The political, social, medical, and computer science world needs to be prepared for the next pandemic virus.

References

1. CLS - trusted market solutions - settlement, processing and data - CLS group. https://www.cls-group.com/. Accessed 09 July 2021
2. Covid-19 (coronavirus disease 2019). http://verywellhealth.com/. Accessed 09 July 2021
3. COVID symptom study. https://covid.joinzoe.com/. Accessed 09 July 2021
4. Data related to coronavirus (COVID-19) - office for national statistics. http://ons.gov.uk/. Accessed 09 July 2021
5. Everywhere you want to be - visa. https://www.visa.co.uk/. Accessed 09 July 2021
6. UK government risk management advice and system guidance. https://www.gov.uk/government/publications/management-of-risk-in-government-framework/. Accessed 09 July 2021
7. Weather forecasting - practical applications. https://www.britannica.com/science/weather-forecasting/Practical-applications/. Accessed 09 July 2021
8. WHO - world health organization. https://www.who.int/. Accessed 09 July 2021
9. Anderson, R.M., Hollingsworth, T.D., Baggaley, R.F., Maddren, R., Vegvari, C.: COVID-19 spread in the UK: the end of the beginning? Lancet **396**(10251), 587–590 (2020). https://doi.org/https://doi.org/10.1016/S0140-6736(20)31689-5. https://www.sciencedirect.com/science/article/pii/S0140673620316895
10. Abu el Ata, N., Perks, M.J.: Solving the Dynamic Complexity Dilemma. Springer, Heidelberg (2014)
11. Khankeh, H., Hosseini, S., Farrokhi, M., et al.: Early warning system models and components in emergency and disaster: a systematic literature review protocol. Syst. Rev. **8**(315), 1–4 (2019)

---

[2] It became public in 2019 it may have been around in some variant form in some creature for many years.

Author Index

Printed in the United States
by Baker & Taylor Publisher Services